The Baby Web

The Directory of Baby-Related Websites

by:
Gretchen Nalley

Published by:

Chestnut Lane
D E S I G N

Chestnut Lane Design, LLC
www.ChestnutLaneDesign.com

The Baby Web

The Directory of Baby-Related Websites

Library of Congress Control Number: 2001119989
ISBN 0-9716372-0-2

Published by:
Chestnut Lane Design, LLC
P.O. Box 1039
Versailles, KY 40383
859-879-1892

books@chestnutlanedesign.com
http://www.ChestnutLaneDesign.com

Table of Contents

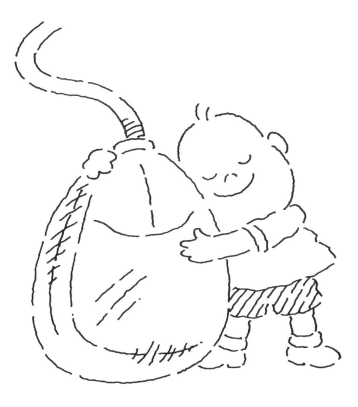

For my son, Zachary
and my husband, Critt.

Special thanks to my parents, Randy and Trudy Barker
and David E. Carter, author and friend.

About the Mother of The Baby Web

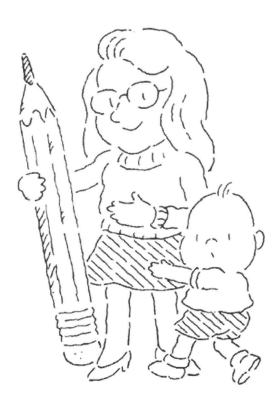

Gretchen Nalley is a computer systems administrator, web designer, full-time mom and now, author. While on maternity leave, she discovered that The World Wide Web included many more informative baby-related Websites than she thought. That led to the birth of this book. She wanted to share these exciting sites with other parents, help them save both time and money and, as much as possible, help make parenthood child's play. She is currently pregnant with her next book.

How to use this book
to get the most out of it.

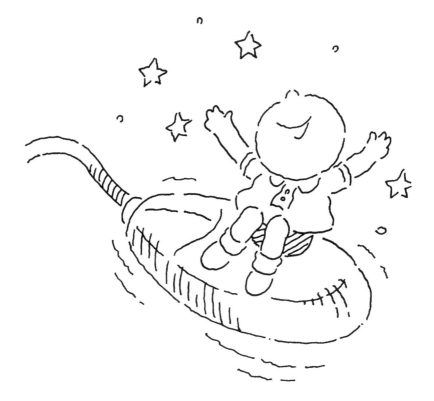

Being a walking encyclopedia of baby-related web sites makes you almost as popular as being a person who can fix computers. I know because I'm both. People ask me questions about toy maker sites with the same regularity as they do about their hard drives, which means often. That's why, when I decided to compile this directory, I wanted to make sure there would be no question on how best to use it. I wanted to make it user-friendly, a no-brainer. I think I've succeeded. Happy surfing!

- All 1,200 web sites are listed both categorically and alphabetically.

- Web sites are segregated into thirteen categories. If you want to know your options, consult this listing.

- All web sites listed categorically have short descriptions of their content.

- If you already know the name of a company, look in the alphabetical index in the back of the book for the address.

- Sites listed with a small book emblem 📖 next to their name indicates that the company offers a catalog.

In Case You Experience A Problem:

All sites were up and running at the publication of this book, and should be still, but if you have a problem, here's what to do:

- Check your spelling and the web site address for .com or .org as they may vary.

- Be sure that the .com is in fact a period and not a comma. Hey, it happens.

- Some sites use www and some do not. Check the address.

- Some sites may really be down temporarily for "repair". Try again later.

Like To Help Write The Next Edition?

If you know of a baby-related web site I haven't included, and you've found to be valuable, e-mail it to me
at books@chestnutlanedesign.com or fill out the "Sug-
gest A Site" form at http://www.chestnutlanedesign.com.
I'd love to share your favorites with other parents.

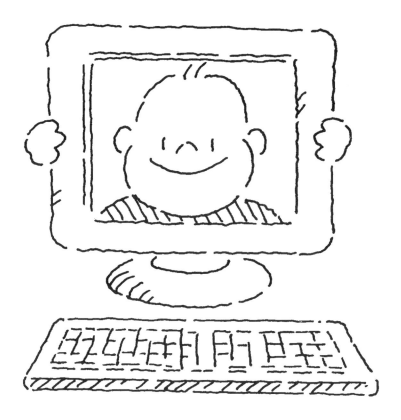

Announcements, Invitations, and Baby Stationary

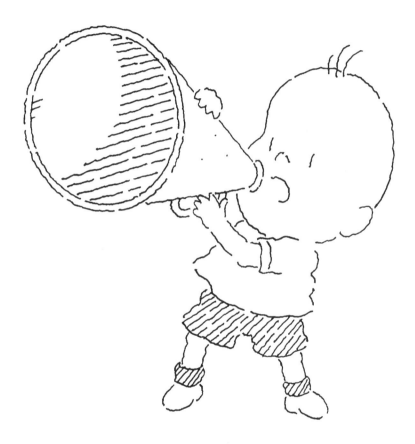

Absolutely Everything.net
Website: http://www.absolutelyeverything.net
Customer Service: 877-243-2465
Announcements, invitations, etc.

Amazing Baby Announcements
Website: http://www.amazingbabyannouncements.com
Customer Service: 888-718-6698
Announcements.

Announcements & More
Website: http://www.announcementsandmore.com
Customer Service: 800-753-1434
Announcements, invitations, and stationary.

A Smart Baby
Website: http://www.asmartbaby.com
Customer Service: 877-310-6647
Educational toys, gifts, videos, books, and announcements.

Babies' N' Bells
Website: http://www.babiesnbells.com
Customer Service: 866-499-BABY
Announcements and invitations.

Baby Bag Online
Website: http://www.babybag.com
Customer Service: 949-388-5257
Baby gear, announcements, pregnancy, parenting, feeding, safety.

Car Brook Publishing
Website: http://www.carbrook.com
Customer Service: 800-201-6231
Announcements in unique sports & collectible cards.

Carson Enterprises Inc.
Website: http://www.ejcarson.com
Customer Service: 800-995-2288
Hershey chocolates wrapped in announcements.

Celebrate that Baby
Website: http://www.celebratethatbaby.com
Customer Service: Ireland
Hand illustrated announcements.

Chocolate Tree
Website: http://www.thechocolatetree.com/birthannouncements
Customer Service: online form
Customized candy bar baby announcements.

Classic Card Co
Website: http://www.classiccard.com
Customer Service: 800-628-0583
Customized announcements and invitations.

Cuscraft 📖
Website: http://www.cuscraft.com
Customer Service: 888-533-BABY
Birth announcements and clothing.

Custom Favors
Website: http://www.customfavors.com/arrivals.htm
Customer Service: 916-771-9151 Fax: 508-526-3054
Candy bars wrapped in a birth announcement.

Daily Diaper, The
Website: http://www.thedailydiaper.com
Customer Service: 866-434-9988
Announcements sent via the website.

Good Buddy Notes
Website: http://www.goodbuddynotes.com
Customer Service: 866-GDBUDDY
Announcements.

Great Announcements
Website: http://www.greatannouncements.com
Customer Service: 888-888-0006
Announcements.

Happy Stork
Website: http://www.happystork.com
Customer Service: 913-696-1366 Fax: 913-696-1286
Announcements.

Imagine Printing
Website: http://www.imagineprinting.com
Customer Service: 888-838-7858
Birth announcements.

Impress In Print
Website: http://www.impressinprint.com
Customer Service: 800-804-1960 Fax: 480-502-1386
Announcements.

J Bink
Website: http://www.jbink.com
Customer Service: 412-825-9442
Announcements.

Kamrya in Print
Website: http://www.partyinvitations.com
Customer Service: 770-682-6015
Announcments and invitations.

Literary Baby
Website: http://www.literarybaby.com
Customer Service: customerservice@literarybaby.com
Announcements.

Little Miracles Invitations
Website: http://www.littlemiracles.invitations.com
Customer Service: 800-491-1139
Announcements.

Moosie Wrapper
Website: http://www.moosiewrapper.com
Customer Service: 800-876-8044
Candy bar announcements.

My Baby Connection
Website: http://www.mybabyconnection.com
Customer Service: webmaster@mybabyconnection.com
Announcements, clothing, gifts, books, and much more.

My Baby Shops
Website: http://www.mybabyshops.com
Customer Service: dawn@mybabyshops.com
Announcements, clothing, gifts, food, and much more.

New Baby
Website: http://www.123gold.com/newbaby
Customer Service: 888-804-8555
Candy bar announcements.

New Baby Announcements
Website: http://www.newbabyannouncements.com
Customer Service: 800-657-6404 ext. 33
Announcements.

New Beginnings
Website: http://www.yournewbeginnings.com
Customer Service: 800-573-2049
Announcments.

Painted Hearts and Friends
Website: http://www.paintedhearts.com
Customer Service: 800-328-4301
Announcments.

Paper Alley
Website: http://www.paperalley.com
Customer Service: 866-56-PAPER
Announcements.

Personalized Baby Gifts
Website: http://www.personalizedbabygifts.com
Customer Service: service@personalizedbabygifts.com
Announcements and gifts.

Picture Perfect Baby
Website: http://www.pictureperfectbaby.com
Customer Service: 877-621-BABY Fax: 919-469-3490
Announcements, baby names, and gifts.

Precious You
Website: http://www.preciousyou.com
Customer Service: 888-371-1888
Announcements.

Preemie Store and More, The
Website: http://www.preemie.com
Customer Service: 800-755-4852
Preemie clothing.

Print Patch
Website: http://www.printpatch.com
Customer Service: 561-790-7719
Announcements.

SMAC Greetings
Website: http://www.smacgreetings.com
Customer Service: 972-962-6062 Fax: 973-962-6069
Customized announcements.

Stork Avenue
Website: http://www.storkavenue.com
Customer Service: 800-861-5437
Announcements and gifts.

Stork Delivers, The
Website: http://www.thestorkdelivers.com
Customer Service: 800-94-BABYS
Gift baskets, bedding, and announcements.

This Baby of Mine
Website: http://www.thisbabyofmine.com
Customer Service: 877-572-6427 Fax: 775-239-1944
Announcements, bedding, books, clothing, care, toys.

Unique Wrappings
Website: http://www.cheerfullychocolate.com
Customer Service: 866-737-5860
Candy bar announcements.

Warm Fuzzys
Website: http://www.warmfuzzys.net/baby.htm
Customer Service: 419-824-7844
Personalized bedding, and announcements.

Wee Snuggles
Website: http://www.weesnuggles.com
Customer Service: 866-665-8631
Announcements and gifts.

We Print Today
Website: http://www.we-print-today.com
Customer Service: 866-744-9444
Announcements.

World Wide Birth Announcements
Website: http://www.greatannouncements.com
Customer Service: 888-304-4646
Announcements.

Baby Care Products

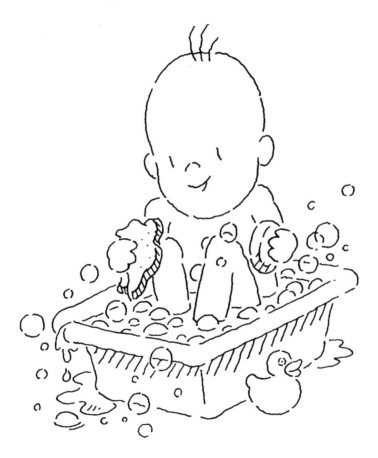

ABC Baby
Website: http://abcbaby.org
Customer Service: mail@abcbaby.org
Baby products guide

ABC Development Inc.
Website: http://www.abc-development.com
Customer Service: 888-222-3053
Baby care, feeding, and toys.

Able Baby
Website: http://www.ablebaby.com
Customer Service: ablebaby@aol.com
Baby care, safety, furniture, videos and toys.

Alternative Baby
Website: http://www.alternativebaby.com
Customer Service: 800-469-1126
Baby care, baby gear, clothing, pregnancy, gift baskets, and toys.

Avent America, Inc.
Website: http://www.aventamerica.com
Customer Service: 800-542-8368
Bottles, breast pumps. skin care, pacifiers, and more.

Babies Planet
Website: http://www.thebabiesplanet.com
Customer Service: susan@babiesplanet.com
Parenting, baby care, health, pregnancy, baby food and names.

Babies-R-Us
Website: http://www.babiesrus.com
Customer Service: 800-BABYRUS
Everything baby- Baby Superstore.

Baby Abby
Website: http://www.babyabby.com
Customer Service: 800-972-7357 Fax: 303-777-6117
Baby care products, clothing, maternity, gifts, safety, and books.

Baby Bag Online
Website: http://www.babybag.com
Customer Service: 949-388-5257
Baby gear, announcements, pregnancy, parenting, feeding, safety.

Baby Best Buy
Website: http://www.babybestbuy.com
Customer Service: 877-BABY-BUY
Baby care, bedding, feeding, and nursing.

Baby Buddy
Website: http://www.babybuddy.com
Customer Service: 877-382-1010
Baby care and safety.

Baby Bunz
Website: http://www.babybunz.com
Customer Service: 800-676-4559 Fax: 360-354-1203
Baby care, clothing, bedding, toys, books, and feeding.

Baby Catalog of America
Website: http://babycatalog.com
Customer Service: 800-PLAYPEN
Baby care, baby gear, furniture, toys, and feeding.

Baby Catalogue, The 📖
Website: http://www.thebabycatalogue.com
Customer Service: London
Clothing, feeding, baby gear, baby care, bedding, safety, and toys.

Baby Concepts
Website: http://www.babyconcepts.com
Customer Service: info@babyconcepts.com
Baby care, clothing, feeding, books, and gifts.

Baby Corner, The
Website: http://www.thebabycorner.com
Customer Service: 812-867-3759
Baby care, pregnancy, parenting, gear, clothing, toys, furniture.

Baby Daily
Website: http://www.babydaily.com
Customer Service: 847-556-2300 Fax: 847-424-9821
Parenting, pregnancy, breastfeeding, and baby care.

Baby Lane
Website: http://www.thebabylane.com
Customer Service: 888-387-0019
Toys, baby care, and baby gear.

Baby Net Center
Website: http://www.babynetcenter.com
Customer Service: online form
Books, clothing, bedding, baby care, feeding, baby gear, and gifts.

Baby News Online
Website: http://www.babynewsonline.com
Customer Service: 866-437-BABY
Baby care, bedding, baby gear, fedding, health and safety.

Baby Online
Website: http://www.babyonline.com
Customer Service: London
Baby care, parenting, feeding, and toys.

Baby Secrets Online
Website: http://www.babysecretsonline.com
Customer Service: 877-818-4800
Baby care and gifts.

Baby Supermall
Website: http://www.babysupermall.com
Customer Service: online form
Baby care, feeding, toys, bedding, gifts, clothing, and safety.

Baby Universe
Website: http://www.babyuniverse.com
Customer Service: 877-615-BABY Fax: 954-523-9881
Health/Safety, feeding, books, baby care, bedding, toys, clothing.

Baby University
Website: http://www.carolinababy.com
Customer Service: dawn@babyuniversity.com
Baby care, pregnancy, parenting, health/safety, and baby names.

Baby's Abode
Website: http://www.babysabode.com
Customer Service: 866-4BBABODE
Toys, baby care, and bedding.

Baby's First Massage
Website: http://www.babysfirstmassage.com
Customer Service: 937-433-5000
Baby care.

Baby's Heaven
Website: http://www.babysheaven.com
Customer Service: 866-343-2836
Gifts, toys, bedding, safety, baby care, and baby gear.

BabyAge.com
Website: http://www.babyage.com
Customer Service: 800-BABYAGE
Health/Safety, bedding, baby gear, feeding, baby care, and gifts.

Babyking
Website: http://babyking.com
Customer Service: 800-424-BABY
Toys, gifts, feeding, clothing, and baby care.

Babyworks
Website: http://www.babyworks.com
Customer Service: 800-422-2910
Feeding, toys, baby care, bedding, and clothing.

Balmex
Website: http://www.balmex.com
Customer Service: 800-245-1040
Baby care products.

Bambini Soul
Website: http://www.bambinisoul.com
Customer Service: 212-929-4365 Fax: 212-633-7033
Baby skin care products.

Bareware
Website: http://bareware.net
Customer Service: 877-9 DIAPER
Baby care, clothing, toys, pregnancy, and baby gear.

Basic Comfort
Website: http://www.basiccomfort.com
Customer Service: 800-456-8687
Health/Safety, baby care, clothing, and bedding.

Basically Baby
Website: http://weeshop.com
Customer Service: 888-254-8780
Bedding, baby care, clothing, and pregnancy.

Born To Love 📖
Website: http://www.borntolove.com
Customer Service: 905-725-2559
Everything diapers.

Calidou
Website: http://www.calidou.com
Customer Service: 800-955-2843
Baby care products.

Character Products
Website: http://www.characterproducts.com
Customer Service: online form
Popular character products.

Cloth Diaper.com
Website: http://www.clothdiaper.com
Customer Service: 877-215-9004
Cloth diapers.

Company Store, The
Website: http://www.thecompanystore.com
Customer Service: 800-323-8000
Toys, baby care, clothing, and bedding.

Cuddly Bub
Website: http://www.cuddlybub.com
Customer Service: Australia
Cute cloth diapers.

Davies Gate 📖
Website: http://www.daviesgate.com
Customer Service: 888-398-9887
Baby care products.

E Baby Station
Website: http://ebabystation.com
Customer Service: 706-863-4452 Fax: 706-863-4452
Gifts, bedding, toys, baby care, baby gear, clothing, pregnancy.

E Baby Superstore
Website: http://www.ebabysuperstore.com
Customer Service: 877-253-7717 Fax: 425-357-1856
Toys, health/safety, baby gear, books/music, baby care.

Earth Baby
Website: http://www.earthbaby.com
Customer Service: 877-602-6800
Baby care, books/music, and clothing.

Eco Baby 📖
Website: http://www.ecobaby.com
Customer Service: 800-596-7450
Pregnancy, bedding, books/music, clothing, and baby care.

Express Baby
Website: http://www.expressbaby.com
Customer Service: 800-600-0410
Feeding, baby gear, gifts, health/safety, baby care, gear, bedding.

Garden Lane
Website: http://www.gardenlane.com
Customer Service: 888-388-7885
Baby care and bedding.

Gentle Mom
Website: http://www.gentlemom.com
Customer Service: 877-833-BABY
Baby care, baby gear, books/music, and parenting.

Gerber
Website: http://www.gerber.com
Customer Service: 800-4GERBER
Baby care products and baby food.

Goodnites
Website: http://www.goodnites.com
Customer Service: 920-721-2553 Fax: 920-721-2035
Disposable, absorbant underpants and parenting tips.

Huggies
Website: http://www.huggies.com
Customer Service: 800-544-1847
Diapers

Huggies Club
Website: http://www.huggiesclub.com
Customer Service: 800-544-1847
Diapers

Huggies Supreme
Website: http://www.parentstages.com
Customer Service: 800-544-1847
Diapers and parenting tips.

I Baby Doc
Website: http://www.ibabydoc.com
Customer Service: 888-758-0272
Baby care, baby gear, health/safety, and gifts.

Johnson & Johnson
Website: http://www.jnj.com
Customer Service: 800-526-3967
Baby care products.

Johnson's Baby Products
Website: http://www.johnsonsbaby.com
Customer Service: 800-526-3967
Baby care products.

Kalencom Corp.
Website: http://www.kalencom.com
Customer Service: 800-344-6699
Diapers, nursery, stroller, and other bags.

Kids II
Website: http://www.kidsii.com
Customer Service: 770-751-0442
Toys, nursery, bath, bouncers, travel.

Leachco
Website: http://www.leachco.com
Customer Service: 800-525-1050
Baby care, safety, nursing, baby gear accessories, and nursery.

Luv n' Care
Website: http://www.luvncare.com
Customer Service: 888-LUVNCARE
Baby care, nursery, and toys.

Luvs
Website: http://www.luvs.com
Customer Service: 888-NO-LEAKS
Diapers

Meijer Baby Club
Website: http://www.meijer.com/babyclub
Customer Service: 800-543-3704
Baby care, toys, bedding, pregnancy, feeding, and more.

Mother-Ease
Website: http://www.motherease.com.com
Customer Service: online form
Diapers .

Mustela USA
Website: http://www.mustela.com
Customer Service: 800-422-2987
Baby skin care.

Natural Mom
Website: http://www.naturalmom.com
Customer Service: 608-242-0200
Health, pregnancy, books, and bath care.

Naturopathica.com
Website: http://www.naturopathica.com
Customer Service: 800-669-7618
Baby care.

Nest Mom
Website: http://www.nestmom.com
Customer Service: 301-824-6378
Baby gear, care, and clothing.

Nursery Bright
Website: http://www.nurserybright.com
Customer Service: 877-BABY-959
Baby care, furniture, bedding, safety, clothing and gear.

One Step Ahead 📖
Website: http://www.onestepahead.com
Customer Service: 800-274-8440
Clothing, baby care, gear, safety, pregnancy, and more.

Pampers
Website: http://www.pampers.com
Customer Service: 800-PAMPERS
Diapers and parenting.

Pampering Boutique
Website: http://www.pamperingboutique.com
Customer Service: 765-449-8514 Fax: same
Baby care, gifts, and clothing.

Preemie Store and More, The 📖
Website: http://www.preemie.com
Customer Service: 800-755-4852
Preemie clothing.

Pregnancy
Website: http://www.women.com/pregnancy
Customer Service: online form
Parenting, pregnancy, babycare, and safety.

Prince Lionheart
Website: http://www.princelionheart.com
Customer Service: 800-544-1132 Fax: 805-982-9442
Bedding, baby care, and safety.

Pull Ups
Website: http://www.pullups.com
Customer Service: online form
Baby care and parenting.

Pump In Style
Website: http://www.pumpinstyle.com
Customer Service: 877-9-DIAPER Fax: 250-336-8848
Nursing, maternity, baby care, toys, clothing, etc.

Red Calliope
Website: http://www.redcalliope.com
Customer Service: 800-421-0526
Safety, bedding, maternity, and baby care.

Rich Frog 📖
Website: http://www.richfrog.com
Customer Service: webinfo@richfrog.com
Toys, gifts, and baby care.

Royal Nursery, The
Website: http://www.newborngifts.com
Customer Service: 858 450 1917
Gifts, music, baby care, bedding, clothing, etc.

Royal Velvet
Website: http://www.royalvelvet.com
Customer Service: 800-476-7112
Baby care and bedding.

Sassy
Website: http://www.sassybaby.com
Customer Service: 800-323-6336
Toys, baby care, feeding, and baby gear.

Shower Baby
Website: http://www.showerbaby.com
Customer Service: 800-945-2429
Baby care.

Sure Baby
Website: http://www.surebaby.com
Customer Service: customercare@surebaby.com
Pregnancy, gifts, and baby care.

Target Lullaby Club
Website: http://www.target.com
Customer Service: 800-888-9333
Everything baby.

This Baby of Mine
Website: http://www.thisbabyofmine.com
Customer Service: 877-572-6427 Fax: 775-239-1944
Announcements, bedding, books, clothing, care, toys.

TL Care
Website: http://www.tlcare.com
Customer Service: online form
Baby care, parenting, and nursing products.

Toys R Us
Website: http://www.toysrus.com
Customer Service: 800-TOYS-R-Us
Toys, feeding, baby care, gear,bedding/furniture, books/music.

Wee Bees
Website: http://www.weebees.com
Customer Service: 877-933-2337
Diapers.

You and Your Child
Website: http://www.tesco.com/youandyourchild
Customer Service: UK
Pregnancy, parenting, feeding, and baby care.

Baby Food and Feeding Supplies.

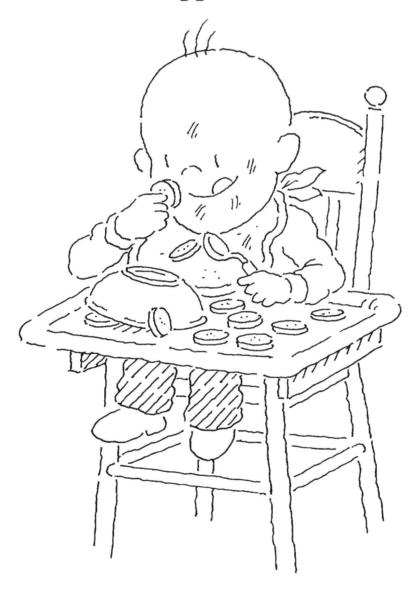

ABC Development Inc.
Website: http://www.abc-development.com
Customer Service: 888-222-3053
Baby care, feeding, and toys.

Ansa
Website: http://www.theansacompany.com
Customer Service: 918-687-1664
Baby bottles, teethers, rattles, cups, etc.

Avent America, Inc.
Website: http://www.aventamerica.com
Customer Service: 800-542-8368
Bottles, breast pumps, skin care, and pacifiers.

Babies-R-Us
Website: http://www.babiesrus.com
Customer Service: 800-BABYRUS
Everything baby- Baby Superstore.

Babies Today
Website: http://babiestoday.com
Customer Service: 847-556-2300 Fax: 847-424-9821
Pregnancy, breastfeeding/ feeding your baby.

Babies Planet
Website: http://www.thebabiesplanet.com
Customer Service: susan@babiesplanet.com
Parenting, baby care, health, pregnancy, baby food and names.

Baby Bag Online
Website: http://www.babybag.com
Customer Service: 949-388-5257
Baby gear, announcements, pregnancy, parenting, feeding, safety.

Baby Best Buy
Website: http://www.babybestbuy.com
Customer Service: 877-BABY-BUY
Bedding, baby care, feeding, and nursing.

Baby Bjorn
Website: http://www.babybjorn.com
Customer Service: 800-593-5522
Baby gear, toys, feeding, and baby care.

Baby Bottle
Website: http://www.babybottle.org
Customer Service: webmaster@babybottle.org
Feeding and safety tips.

Baby Bunz
Website: http://www.babybunz.com
Customer Service: 800-676-4559 Fax: 360-354-1203
Baby care, clothing, bedding, toys, books, and feeding.

Baby Catalog of America
Website: http://babycatalog.com
Customer Service: 800-PLAYPEN
Baby care, baby gear, furniture, toys, and feeding.

Baby Catalogue, The 📖
Website: http://www.thebabycatalogue.com
Customer Service: London
Clothing, feeding, baby gear, baby care, bedding, safety, and toys.

Baby Concepts
Website: http://www.babyconcepts.com
Customer Service: info@babyconcepts.com
Baby care, clothing, feeding, books, and gifts.

Baby Cyberstore
Website: http://www.babycyberstore.com
Customer Service: 757-369-0254 Fax: 757-369-0256
Bedding, baby gear, toys, and feeding.

Baby Foods
Website: http://www.nestle.com/in_your_life/baby_foods
Customer Service: online form
Baby food and cereal.

Baby Gifts 4 Less
Website: http://www.babygifts-4less.com
Customer Service: 877-378-4411
Baby gear, safety, bedding, toys, feeding, maternity, and gifts.

Baby Land / Baby Land Kids Room
Website: http://www.babyland-kidsroom.com
Customer Service: 888-316-8952
Furniture, baby gear, feeding, safety, and gifts.

Baby Love Products 📖
Website: http://www.babyloveproducts.com
Customer Service: 780-672-1763
Baby gear and breastfeeding supplies.

Baby Mountain
Website: http://www.babymountain.com
Customer Service: mail@babymountain.com
Announcements, clothing, baby food, names, toys, safety, bedding.

Baby Navigator
Website: http://www.babynavigator.com
Customer Service: online form
Baby gear, nursery, safety, feeding, baby care, toys, books, etc.

Baby Needs
Website: http://www.babyneeds.com
Customer Service: 800-672-5313
Parenting, feeding, health and safety.

Baby Net Center
Website: http://www.babynetcenter.com
Customer Service: online form
Books/music, clothing, gifts, bedding, feeding, baby care, and gear.

Baby News Online
Website: http://www.babynewsonline.com
Customer Service: 866-437-BABY
Bedding, baby gear, baby care, feeding, health/safety.

Baby oh Baby
Website: http://www.baby-oh-baby.com
Customer Service: 800-825-4901
Feeding and gifts.

Baby Online
Website: http://www.babyonline.com
Customer Service: London
Baby care, parenting, toys, and feeding.

Baby Store
Website: http://www.baby-store.net
Customer Service: 877-378-4411
Feeding, safety, pregnancy, bedding, and baby gear.

Baby Supermall
Website: http://www.babysupermall.com
Customer Service: online form
Baby care, feeding, toys, bedding, gifts, clothing, and safety.

Baby Tips
Website: http://www.babytips.co.uk
Customer Service: UK
Feeding, health and safety, pregnancy, and parenting.

Baby Universe
Website: http://www.babyuniverse.com
Customer Service: 877-615-BABY Fax: 954-523-9881
Health/Safety, feeding, books, baby care, bedding, toys, clothing.

BabyAge.com
Website: http://www.babyage.com
Customer Service: 800-BABYAGE
Health/Safety, bedding, baby gear, feeding, baby care, and gifts.

Babyking
Website: http://babyking.com
Customer Service: 800-424-BABY
Toys, gifts, feeding, clothing, and baby care.

Babynet Center
Website: http://www.babynetcenter.com
Customer Service: online form
Books/music, clothing, feeding, baby gear, toys, bedding, gifts.

Babyworks
Website: http://www.babyworks.com
Customer Service: 800-422-2910
Feeding, toys, baby care, bedding, and clothing.

Beechnut
Website: http://www.beechnut.com
Customer Service: 314-877-7145
Baby food.

Carnation
Website: http://www.carnationbaby.com
Customer Service: 800-CARNATION
Baby food and formula, parenting, and pregnancy.

Character Products
Website: http://www.characterproducts.com
Customer Service: online form
Popular character prodcuts.

Child Birth
Website: http://www.childbirth.org
Customer Service: 502-897-7664
Pregnancy and feeding.

Dr. Brown's Baby Bottle
Website: http://www.handi-craft.com
Customer Service: 800-778-9001
Natural flow baby bottles.

Earth's Best
Website: http://www.earthsbest.com
Customer Service: 303-530-5300 Fax: 303-381-1349
Baby food, cereals, juices, etc.

Enfamil
Website: http://www.enfamil.com
Customer Service: 800 BABY-123
Baby formula and parenting guides.

Express Baby
Website: http://www.expressbaby.com
Customer Service: 800-600-0410
Feeding, baby gear, health/safety, clothing, baby care, bedding.

Gerber Feeding
Website: http://www.gerber.com
Customer Service: 800-4GERBER
Baby food.

Heinz Baby
Website: http://www.heinzbaby.com
Customer Service: 800-565-2100
Baby food.

MAWS
Website: http://www.maws-usa.com
Customer Service: 888-570-6297 Fax: 925-930-7792
Bottles

Mead Johnson Nutritionals
Website: http://www.meadjohnson.com
Customer Service: 812-439-5000
Health and baby food.

Meijer Baby Club
Website: http://www.meijer.com/babyclub
Customer Service: 800-543-3704
Feeding, bedding, baby care, pregnancy, toys, and baby gear.

My Baby Shops
Website: http://www.mybabyshops.com
Customer Service: dawn@mybabyshops.com
Announcements, clothing, gifts, food, and much more.

Neat Solutions Inc.
Website: http://www.tabletopper.com
Customer Service: 888-888-4779 Fax: 704-895-4409
Baby food.

Nestle
Website: http://www.nestle.com
Customer Service: 818-549-6818 Fax: 818-549-6330
Baby food.

Playtex Baby
Website: http://www.playtexbaby.com
Customer Service: 800-222-0453
Baby feeding and baby care.

Preemie Store and More, The 📖
Website: http://www.preemie.com
Customer Service: 800-755-4852
Preemie clothing.

Safety 1st
Website: http://www.safety1st.com
Customer Service: 800-723-3065
Safety, baby gear, and baby food.

Sassy
Website: http://www.sassybaby.com
Customer Service: 800-323-6336
Toys, baby care, feeding, and baby gear.

Similac
Website: http://www.similac.com
Customer Service: 800-227-5767
Parenting and baby formula.

Sip and Snap
Website: http://www.sipandsnap.com
Customer Service: 800-742-3104 Fax: 909-357-9580
Sippy cups.

Super Baby Food
Website: http://www.superbabyfood.com
Customer Service: 866-BABY-BOOK
Baby food book; guide to making baby food.

Toys R Us
Website: http://www.toysrus.com
Customer Service: 800-TOYS-R-Us
Toys, feeding, baby care, gear,bedding/furniture, books/music.

Vegetarian Baby
Website: http://www.vegetarianbaby.com
Customer Service: editor@vegetarianbaby.com
Baby food.

Vegetarian Resource Group
Website: http://www.vrg.org/recipes/babyfood.html
Customer Service: 410-366-8343
Baby food.

Very Best Baby
Website: http://www.verybestbaby.com
Customer Service: 800-456-6035
Health, food, parenting, and more.

You and Your Child
Website: http://www.tesco.com/youandyourchild
Customer Service: UK
Pregnancy, parenting, feeding, and baby care.

Your Amazing Baby
Website: http://www.amazingbaby.com
Customer Service: kellyr@amazingbaby.com
Parenting, safety, and feeding.

Baby Gear and Accessories

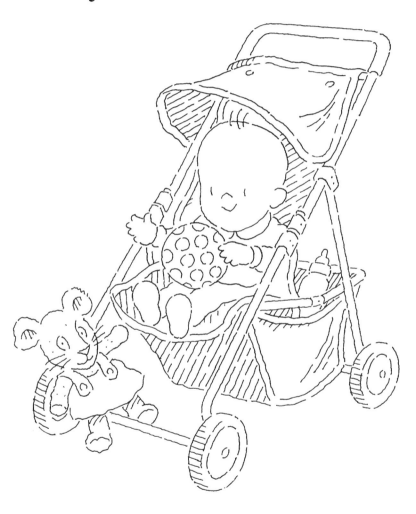

Alternative Baby
Website: http://www.alternativebaby.com
Customer Service: 800-469-1126
Baby care, baby gear, clothing, pregnancy, gift baskets, and toys.

Aprica USA, Inc.
Website: http://www.apricausa.com
Customer Service: 310- 639-6387
Baby gear and parenting.

Arm's Reach
Website: http://www.armsreach.com
Customer Service: 800-954-9353
Baby gear and co-sleeper cribs.

Attachments 📖
Website: http://www.attachmentscatalog.com
Customer Service: 800-873-5023
Baby gear, gifts, toys, books/music, and pregnancy.

B.O.B. Sport Utility Stroller 📖
Website: http://www.bobtrailers.com
Customer Service: 800-893-2447
Baby gear.

Babies-R-Us
Website: http://www.babiesrus.com
Customer Service: 800-BABYRUS
Baby gear, gifts, toys, bedding, books/music, clothing, baby care.

Baby Abby
Website: http://www.babyabby.com
Customer Service: 800-972-7357 Fax: 303-777-6117
Baby care, baby gear, clothing, books/music, gifts, health/safety.

Baby Bag Online
Website: http://www.babybag.com
Customer Service: 949-388-5257
Baby gear, announcements, pregnancy, parenting, feeding, safety.

Baby B'air
Website: http://www.babybair.com
Customer Service: 800-417-5228
Baby B'air flight vest for babies that fly in airplanes.

Baby Bazaar
Website: http://www.babybazaar.com
Customer Service: 877-543-7186
Clothing, baby gear, toys, gifts, and furniture.

Baby Bjorn
Website: http://www.babybjorn.com
Customer Service: 800-593-5522
Baby gear, toys, feeding, and baby care.

Baby Bundler Inc.
Webs ite: http://www.babybundler.com
Cus tomer Service: 503-293-8503
Baby gear.

Baby Cam, The
Website: http://www.thebabycam.com
Customer Service: 800-816-9883
Hidden cameras to monitor nannies and babysitters.

Baby Care
Website: http://babycare-sa.com
Customer Service: 866-343-2836
Baby gear, bedding, gifts, nursing, toys, and pregnancy.

Baby Catalog of America
Website: http://babycatalog.com
Customer Service: 800-PLAYPEN
Baby gear, furniture, baby care, toys, and feeding.

Baby Catalogue, The 📖
Website: http://www.thebabycatalogue.com
Customer Service: London
Clothing, feeding, baby gear, baby care, bedding, toys, and safety.

Baby Center
Website: http://www.babycenter.com
Customer Service: online form
Parenting, pregnancy, announcements, baby gear, safety, etc.

Baby Cleanseat
Website: http://www.babycleanseat.cc
Customer Service: 877-655-8384
Baby seat for public shopping carts and high chairs.

Baby Comfort
Website: http://www.basiccomfort.com
Customer Service: 800-456-8687
Baby comfort strap for shopping carts.

Baby Corner, The
Website: http://www.thebabycorner.com
Customer Service: 812-867-3759
Baby care, pregnancy, parenting, bedding, gear, clothing, toys.

Baby Cyberstore
Website: http://www.babycyberstore.com
Customer Service: 757-369-0254 Fax: 757-369-0256
Bedding, baby gear, toys, feeding, and more.

Baby Elegance, Inc.
Website: http://www.babyelegance.com
Customer Service: 818-349-1442 Fax: 818-361-6695
Baby gear.

Baby Gear Review
Website: http://www.babygearreview.com
Customer Service: 408-738-7300 Fax: 408-737-2803
Baby gear reviews.

Baby Gifts 4 Less
Website: http://www.babygifts-4less.com
Customer Service: 877-378-4411
Baby gear, safety, furniture, toys, feeding, maternity, and gifts.

Baby Hut
Website: http://www.babyhut.com
Customer Service: 813-907-8928
Baby gear, bedding, and safety.

Baby Jogger
Website: http://www.babyjogger.com
Customer Service: 800-241-1848
Baby jogging strollers and accessories.

Baby Land / Baby Land Kids Room
Website: http://www.babyland-kidsroom.com
Customer Service: 888-316-8952
Furniture, baby gear, feeding, safety, and gifts.

Baby Lane
Website: http://www.thebabylane.com
Customer Service: 888-387-0019
Toys, baby care, and baby gear.

Baby Love Products 📖
Website: http://www.babyloveproducts.com
Customer Service: 780-672-1763
Baby gear and breastfeeding supplies.

Baby n' Mom
Website: http://www.baby-n-mom.com
Customer Service: webmaster@best-toy-prices.com
Baby names, furniture, clothing, gear, and parenting.

Baby Navigator
Website: http://www.babynavigator.com
Customer Service: online form
Baby gear, nursery, safety, feeding, baby care, toys, books/music.

Baby Net Center
Website: http://www.babynetcenter.com
Customer Service: online form
Books/music, clothing, bedding, baby care, feeding, baby gear.

Baby News Online
Website: http://www.babynewsonline.com
Customer Service: 866-437-BABY
Bedding, baby gear, feeding, baby care, health/safety.

Baby Polar Gear
Website: http://www.babypolargear.com
Customer Service: 866-bby-gear
Baby gear.

Baby Products Online
Website: http://www.babyproductsonline.com
Customer Service: 626-914-9905
Gifts, toys, bedding, and baby gear.

Baby See Shell
Website: http://www.babyseeshell.com
Customer Service: 800-223-0686 (code 88)
Baby gear.

Baby Shower Mall
Website: http://www.babyshowermall.com
Customer Service: 888-831-6243
Baby gear, bedding, and gifts.

Baby Style
Website: http://www.babystyle.com
Customer Service: 877-ESTYLES
Bedding, baby gear, gifts, toys, and clothing.

Baby Toy Town
Website: http://www.babytoytown.com
Customer Service: 626-288-6220
Gifts, baby gear, bedding, and toys.

Baby Trend Corp
Website: http://www.babytrend.com
Customer Service: 800-328-7363
Baby gear.

Baby Warehouse
Website: http://www.thebabywarehouse.com
Customer Service: 877-450-2323
Bedding, baby gear, gifts, toys, and clothing.

Baby's Away
Website: http://www.babysaway.com
Customer Service: 800-571-0077
Baby and child supply rental service.

Baby's Heaven
Website: http://www.babysheaven.com
Customer Service: 866-343-2836
Gifts, toys, bedding, health/safety, baby care, and baby gear.

BabyAge.com
Website: http://www.babyage.com
Customer Service: 800-BABYAGE
Health/safety, bedding, baby gear, feeding, baby care, and gifts.

Babynet Center
Website: http://www.babynetcenter.com
Customer Service: online form
Books/music, clothing, feeding, baby gear, toys, bedding, and gifts.

Baby's Image
Website: http://www.babysimage.com
Customer Service: 800-972-2202
Baby gear.

Bareware
Website: http://bareware.net
Customer Service: 877-9 DIAPER
Baby gear, baby care, pregnancy, toys, and clothing.

Bebe Sounds
Website: http://www.bebesounds.com
Customer Service: 800-233-1196 Fax: 212-736-6762
Baby gear, books/music.

Bed Wetting Store
Website: http://www.bedwettingstore.com
Customer Service: 800-214-9605
Baby gear.

Bob Strollers
Website: http://www.bobstrollers.com
Customer Service: 800-893-2447
Bicycle trailers and strollers/joggers.

Britax
Website: http://www.childseat.com
Customer Service: 888-427-4829
Baby gear.

Bundle Me
Website: http://www.bundleme.com
Customer Service: 800-987-6828
Baby buntings.

CPSC
Website: http://www.cpsc.gov
Customer Service: 800-638-2772
Baby gear and parenting.

Canada Baby Works
Website: http://www.canadababyworks.com
Customer Service: 877-531-BABY
Clothing, baby care, toys, pregnancy, and baby gear.

Character Products
Website: http://www.characterproducts.com
Customer Service: online forms
Popular character products.

Cherish & Joy Kidstuff
Website: http://www.cherish&joy.com
Customer Service: 888-745-5922
Baby gear, bedding, and clothing.

Cherished Moments
Website: http://www.cherishedmoments.com
Customer Service: 713-957-2764 Fax: 713-957-2764
Toys, bedding, parenting, baby gear and names.

Chicco USA
Website: http://www.chiccousa.com
Customer Service: 877-424-4226
Baby gear and toys.

Child Seat
Website: http://www.childseat.com
Customer Service: 704-409-1700
Baby gear.

Children's Orchard
Website: http://www.childorch.com
Customer Service: 800-999-KIDS
Baby gear, toys, and clothing.

Comfort Living
Website: http://www.baby-store.net
Customer Service: 877-378-4411
Baby gear, toys, health/safety, bedding, pregnancy, feeding.

Cosco Inc.
Website: http://www.coscoinc.com
Customer Service: 800-544-1108
Baby gear and toys.

D.E.X. Products
Website: http://www.dexproducts.com
Customer Service: 800-546-1996
Baby gear and bedding.

E Baby Station
Website: http://ebabystation.com
Customer Service: 706-863-4452 Fax: 706-863-4452
Gifts, bedding, pregnancy, baby care, baby gear, toys, clothing.

E Baby Superstore
Website: http://www.ebabysuperstore.com
Customer Service: 877-253-7717 Fax: 425-357-1856
Toys, health/safety, baby gear, books/music, andbaby care.

EStyle
Website: http://www.estyle.com
Customer Service: 877-ESTYLES
Bedding, toys, clothing, pregnancy, gifts, and baby gear.

Eddie Bauer
Website: http://www.eddiebauer.com
Customer Service: 800-426-8020
Baby gear and clothing.

Emmaljunga
Website: http://www.emmaljunga.com
Customer Service: 800-232-4411
Baby gear.

Evenflo
Website: http://www.carseat.com
Customer Service: 800-233-5921
Baby gear.

Express Baby
Website: http://www.expressbaby.com
Customer Service: 800-600-0410
Feeding, baby gear, health/safety, clothing, bedding, baby care.

Gentle Mom
Website: http://www.gentlemom.com
Customer Service: 877-833-BABY
Baby gear, baby care, books/music, and parenting.

Graco
Website: http://www.graco.com
Customer Service: 800-345-4109
Baby gear.

Graco Baby
Website: http://www.gracobaby.com
Customer Service: 800-345-4109
Baby gear.

Great Beginnings
Website: http://www.childrensfurniture.com
Customer Service: 800-886-7099
Bedding/furniture, baby gear, toys, safety, books/music, and gifts.

Hip Hammock
Website: http://www.hiphammock.com
Customer Service: 203-343-0016
Baby gear.

I Baby Doc
Website: http://www.ibabydoc.com
Customer Service: 888-758-0272
Baby care, baby gear, health/safety, and gifts.

Infantino
Website: http://www.infantino.com
Customer Service: 800-365-8182 Fax: 858-457-0181
Baby gear, bedding, and toys.

Inglesina
Website: http://www.inglesina.com
Customer Service: 877-486-5112
Strollers, Prams, baby seats, table mounted chairs, etc.

Kalencom Corp.
Website: http://www.kalencom.com
Customer Service: 800-344-6699
Diaper, nursery, stroller, and other bags.

Kel-Gar Inc.
Website: http://www.kelgar.com
Customer Service: 800-388-1848 Fax: 972-250-3805
Baby gear.

Kelty Kids
Website: http://www.kelty.com
Customer Service: 800-423-2320 Fax: 800-504-2745
Infant carriers, strollers, accessories.

KidCo Inc.
Website: http://www.kidcoinc.com
Customer Service: 800-553-5529
Strollers, gates, safety, and carriers.

Kiddopotamus
Website: http://www.kiddopotamus.com
Customer Service: 800-772-8339
Strollers, shades, safety.

Kids II
Website: http://www.kidsii.com
Customer Service: 770-751-0442
Toys, nursery, bath, bouncers, travel.

Kolcraft Enterprises
Website: http://www.kolcraft.com
Customer Service: 800-453-7673
Baby gear.

Kool Stop
Website: http://www.koolstop.com
Customer Service: 800-586-3332
Baby gear.

Lamby Nursery Collection
Website: http://www.lamby.com
Customer Service: 800-669-0527
Baby gear accessories and bedding.

Leachco
Website: http://www.leachco.com
Customer Service: 800-525-1050
Bedding, baby care, health/safety, baby gear, and pregnancy.

Lillie Bugs
Website: http://www.lilliebugs.com
Customer Service: 320-769-2347 Fax: 320-769-2347
Baby gear accessories.

Marrott Baby Products
Website: http://www.babyproductsstore.com
Customer Service: service@babyproductsstore.com
Baby gear and safety

Mason, J.
Website: http://www.jmason.com
Customer Service: 800-242-1922
Baby gear.

Maya Wrap
Website: http://www.mayawrap.com
Customer Service: mayawrap@mayawrap.com
Baby gear.

Nest Mom
Website: http://www.nestmom.com
Customer Service: 301-824-6378
Baby gear, care, and clothing.

Nursery Bright
Website: http://www.nurserybright.com
Customer Service: 877-BABY-959
Baby care, furniture, bedding, safety, clothing, and gear.

Nursery Rhymes
Website: http://www.nurseryrhymes.com
Customer Service: 519-743-1321 Fax: 519-743-1681
Baby gear, furniture and bedding, toys, and safety.

Nursing
Website: http://www.russettweb.com/nursing.html
Customer Service: 877-865-9786
Baby gear and nursing information.

One Hot Mama
Website: http://www.one hotmama.com
Customer Service: 800-217-3750
Clothing, nursing, and baby gear.

One Step Ahead
Website: http://www.onestepahead.com
Customer Service: 800-274-8440
Clothing, baby care, gear, safety, pregnancy, and more.

Parenting Concepts
Website: http://www.parentingconcepts.com
Customer Service: 800-727-3683
Baby gear, books/music, parenting, toys, and gifts.

Peg Perego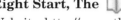
Website: http://www.perego.com
Customer Service: 800-728-2108
Baby gear and toys.

Pregnant Inc.
Website: http://www.pregnantinc.com
Customer Service: 626-288-6220
Bedding, furniture, and baby gear.

Right Start, The
Website: http://www.therightstart.com
Customer Service: 800-LITTLE-1
Books, baby gear, health, safety, and much more.

Safety 1st
Website: http://www.safety1st.com
Customer Service: 800-723-3065
Safety, baby gear, and baby food.

Sassy
Website: http://www.sassybaby.com
Customer Service: 800-323-6336
Toys, baby care, feeding, and baby gear.

Security and More
Website: http://www.securityandmore.com
Customer Service: 800-444-6278
Safety, high tech baby monitors.

Sheep Skin Express
Website: http://www.sheepskinexpress.com
Customer Service: 866-287-8495 Fax: 877-890-7773
Sheep skin products such as rugs and car seat covers.

Smart Choice
Website: http://www.smart-choice.com
Customer Service: 800-444-6278
High tech baby monitors.

Target Lullaby Club
Website: http://www.target.com
Customer Service: 800-888-9333
Everything baby.

Tots in Mind
Website: http://www.totsinmind.com
Customer Service: 800-626-0339
Baby gear.

Tough Traveler
Website: http://www.toughtraveler.com
Customer Service: 800-468-6844
Baby gear.

Toys R Us
Website: http://www.toysrus.com
Customer Service: 800-TOYS-R-Us
Toys, feeding, baby care, gear,bedding/furniture, books/music.

Traveling Tikes
Website: http://www.travelingtikes.com
Customer Service: 877-698-4537
Baby gear.

Tuttibella
Website: http://www.tuttibella.com
Customer Service: 877-279-9391
Bedding, furniture, clothes, toys, baby gear, and more.

UK Mother
Website: http://www.ukmother.com
Customer Service: UK
Pregnancy, health, baby gear.

Vaporeze
Website: http://www.vaporeze.com
Customer Service: 877-343-1241
Waterless vaporizer.

Wee Go
Website: http://www.weego.com
Customer Service: 800-676-0352
Baby gear.

Yahoo
Website: http://shoppingyahoo.com
Customer Service: online form
Furniture, clothing, bedding, baby gear, and more.

Baby Names

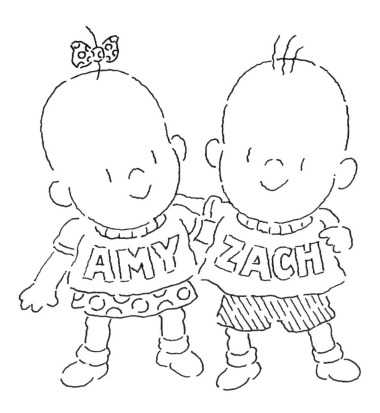

Adorable Baby Gifts
Website: http://www.adorablebabygifts.com
Customer Service: 713-666-0844
Gifts, clothing, and baby names.

Babies Planet
Website: http://www.thebabiesplanet.com
Customer Service: susan@thebabuesplanet.com
Parenting, baby care, health, pregnancy, baby foods and names.

Baby Chatter
Website: http://www.babychatter.com
Customer Service: info@babychatter.com
Baby names, safety, books, and announcements.

Baby Mountain
Website: http://www.babymountain.com
Customer Service: mail@babymountain.com
Announcements, clothing, feeding, names, toys, safety, bedding.

Baby n' Mom
Website: http://www.baby-n-mom.com
Customer Service: webmaster@best-toys-prices.com
Clothing, bedding, parenting, baby names, and baby gear.

Baby Namer
Website: http://www.babynamer.com
Customer Service: editor@babynamer.com
Baby names.

Baby Names
Website: http://www.babynames.com
Customer Service: online form
Baby names.

Baby Names
Website: http://babynames.keepkidshealthy.com
Customer Service: online form
Baby names.

Baby Name Search
Website: http://www.babynamesearch.com
Customer Service: bestobest@usa.net
Baby names.

Baby Outlet
Website: http://www.babyoutlet.com
Customer Service: home@babyoutlet.com
Books/music and baby names.

Baby Zone
Website: http://www.babyzone.com
Customer Service: webmaster@babyzone.com
Baby names, parenting, announcements, and pregnancy.

Carolina Baby
Website: http://www.carolinababy.com
Customer Service: dawn@babyuniversity.com
Baby care, names, pregnancy, parenting, health/safety.

Cherished Moments
Website: http://www.cherishedmoments.com
Customer Service: 713-957-2764 Fax: 713-957-2764
Toys, bedding, parenting, baby gear and names.

E Pregnancy
Website: http://www.epregnancy.com
Customer Service: 925-447-6667 Fax: 925-937-7203
Pregnancy, books, and baby names.

First Names
Website: http://www.zelo.com/firstnames
Customer Service: online form
Baby names.

For Babies
Website: http://www.4babies.com
Customer Service: 510-768-1444
Books, parenting, clothing, safety, and baby names.

I Maternity
Website: http://www.imaternity.com
Customer Service: 800-344-0011
Pregnancy and baby names.

Kabalarians
Website: http://www.kabalarians.com
Customer Service: 604-263-9551 Fax: 604-263-5514
Baby names.

Motherhood Maternity
Website: http://www.motherhood.com
Customer Service: 800-4-MOM-2-BE
Maternity/nursing wear and baby names.

New Baby Name Index
Website: http://www.newbabynameindex.com
Customer Service: nbni@newbabynameindex.com
Baby names.

Picture Perfect Baby
Website: http://www.pictureperfectbaby.com
Customer Service: 877-621-BABY Fax: 919-469-3490
Announcements, baby names, and gifts.

Popular Baby Names
Website: http://www.popularbabynames.com
Customer Service: online form
Baby names, books and music.

Bedding, Furniture, and Nursery Decor.

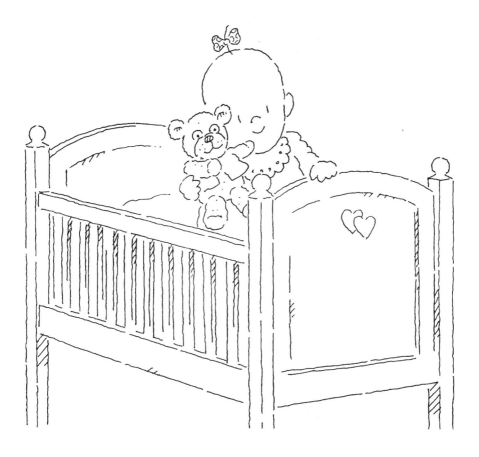

American Blind and Wallpaper Factory
Website: http://www.decoratetoday.com
Cus tomer Service: 800-735-5300
Decorative advicefor baby's room.

American Creative Team, Inc.
Website: http://www.us-act.com
Customer Service: 800-747-5689
Wall hangings, fun wall cling scenes, and toys.

Amy Coe, Inc.
Website: http://www.amycoe.com
Customer Service: 203-221-3050
Baby bedding.

Angel Baby by Legacy
Website: http://www.legacylinens.com
Customer Service: online form
Baby bedding.

Angel Line
Website: http://www.angelline.com
Customer Service: 800-889-8158
Baby bedding.

Arm's Reach
Website: http://www.armsreach.com
Customer Service: 800-954-9353
Baby bedding.

Arrivals Baby Gifts
Website: http://www.arrivalsbabygifts.com
Customer Service: 800-741-0254
Bedding, toys, and gifts.

Babi Italia
Website: http://www.babiitalia.com
Customer Service: 877-440-2224
Baby bedding.

Babies-R-Us
Website: http://www.babiesrus.com
Customer Service: 800-BABYRUS
Baby gear, toys, bedding, clothing, books/music, and gifts.

Baby Ant
Website: http://www.babyant.com
Customer Service: online form
Bedding, health/safety, toys, gifts, and clothing.

Baby Bazaar
Website: http://www.babybazaar.com
Customer Service: 877-543-7186
Bedding, toys, clothing, gifts, and baby gear.

Baby Bedding
Website: http://www.babybedding.com
Customer Service: 800-600-5190
Baby bedding.

Baby Best Buy
Website: http://www.babybestbuy.com
Customer Service: 877-BABY-BUY
Bedding, baby care, feeding, and nursing.

Baby Blankets Etc.
Website: http://www.babyblankets-etc.com
Customer Service: 231-946-3341 Fax: 231-929-9210
Baby blankets.

Baby Box
Website: http://babybox.com
Customer Service: 800-373-8216
Toys, gifts, books/music, clothing, and bedding.

Baby Bunk
Website: http://babybunk.com
Customer Service: 617-323-6539
Co-sleep safely with this bassinet alternative.

Baby Bunz
Website: http://www.babybunz.com
Customer Service: 800-676-4559 Fax: 360-354-1203
Baby care, clothing, bedding, toys, books/music, and feeding.

Baby Care
Website: http://babycare-sa.com
Customer Service: 866-343-2836
Baby gear, bedding, gifts, nursing, toys, and more.

Baby Catalog of America
Website: http://babycatalog.com
Customer Service: 800-PLAYPEN
Baby gear, bedding/furniture, baby care, toys, and feeding.

Baby Catalogue, The 📖
Website: http://www.thebabycatalogue.com
Customer Service: London
Clothing, feeding, baby gear, baby care, bedding, health/safety.

Baby Chatter
Website: http://www.babychatter.com
Customer Service: online form
Names, safety, books, announcements, and bedding.

Baby Corner, The
Website: http://www.thebabycorner.com
Customer Service: 812-867-3759
Baby care, pregnancy, parenting, gear, clothing, toys, bedding.

Baby Cyberstore
Website: http://www.babycyberstore.com
Customer Service: 757-369-0254 Fax: 757-369-0256
Bedding, baby gear, toys, feeding.

Baby Emporio
Website: http://www.babyemporio.com
Customer Service: 800-965-9909
Ookie and kammi dolls, blankets, and soothys.

Baby Estore
Website: http://www.babyestore.com
Customer Service: 866-580-BABY
Breastfeeding supplies, bedding, and gifts.

Baby Express Stores 📖
Website: http://www.babyexpressstores.com
Customer Service: info@babyexpressstores.com
Bedding and furniture.

Baby Gift Idea
Website: http://www.babygiftidea.com
Customer Service: 904-880-2836
Gifts and nursery decor.

Baby Gifts 4 Less
Website: http://www.babygifts-4less.com
Customer Service: 877-378-4411
Baby gear, safety, bedding, toys, feeding, pregnancy, and gifts.

Baby Goodies
Website: http://www.babygoodies.com
Customer Service: 845-658-9808
Gifts and baby blankets.

Baby Hut
Website: http://www.babyhut.com
Customer Service: 813-907-8928
Baby gear, bedding, and safety.

Baby Land
Website: http://www.babyland.com
Customer Service: stork@babyland.com
Announcements, books, and parenting.

Baby Land / Baby Land Kids Room
Website: http://www.babyland-kidsroom.com
Customer Service: 888-316-8952
Bedding, baby gear, feeding, safety, and gifts.

Baby Martex
Website: http://www.babymartex.com
Customer Service: 888-694-2337
Bedding.

Baby n' Mom
Website: http://www.baby-n-mom.com
Customer Service: webmaster@best-toy-prices.com
Baby names, bedding, clothing, baby gear, and parenting.

Baby Navigator
Website: http://www.babynavigator.com
Customer Service: online form
Safety, bedding, feeding, toys, baby care, gear, clothing, and books.

Baby Net Center
Website: http://www.babynetcenter.com
Customer Service: online form
Clothing, bedding, feeding, baby gear, baby care, books, gifts.

Baby News Online
Website: http://www.babynewsonline.com
Customer Service: 866-437-BABY
Bedding, baby gear, baby care, feeding, health/safety.

Baby Paradise
Website: http://www.babyparadise.com
Customer Service: 877-580-8717
Bedding.

Baby Products
Website: http://www.baby-products.com
Customer Service: 303-464-8285 Fax: 303-497-9415
Baby gear, bedding, toys, and gifts.

Baby Shower Mall
Website: http://www.babyshowermall.com
Customer Service: 888-831-6243
Baby gear, bedding, and gifts.

Baby Style
Website: http://www.babystyle.com
Customer Service: 877-ESTYLES
Bedding, toys, clothing, baby gear, baby care.

Baby Supermall
Website: http://www.babysupermall.com
Customer Service: online form
Baby care, feeding, toys, bedding, clothing, health/safety.

Baby Toy Town
Website: http://www.babytoytown.com
Customer Service: 626-288-6220
Toys, bedding, baby gear, and gifts.

Baby Universe
Website: http://www.babyuniverse.com
Customer Service: 877-615-BABY Fax: 954-523-9881
Safety, feeding, books, baby care, gear, toys, bedding and clothing.

Baby's Abode
Website: http://www.babysabode.com
Customer Service: 866-4BBABODE
Toys, baby care, and bedding.

Baby's Dream
Website: http://www.babysdream.com
Customer Service: 800-TEL-CRIB
Bedding.

Baby's Heaven
Website: http://www.babysheaven.com
Customer Service: 866-343-2836
Toys, bedding, health/safety, baby care, gear, gifts.

BabyAge.com
Website: http://www.babyage.com
Customer Service: 800-BABYAGE
Bedding, feeding, baby care, gear, gifts, safety.

Babynet Center
Website: http://www.babynetcenter.com
Customer Service: online form
Books/music, clothing, feeding, bedding, toys, baby gear.

Baby's Room
Website: http://www.babysroom.com
Customer Service: 800-323-4108
Bedding and furniture.

Babyworks
Website: http://www.babyworks.com
Customer Service: 800-422-2910
Feeding, toys, babycare, bedding, clothing.

Badger Basket
Website: http://www.badgerbasket.com
Customer Service: 800-236-1310
Bedding.

Basic Comfort
Website: http://www.basiccomfort.com
Customer Service: 800-456-8687
Bedding, clothing, baby care, and health/safety.

Basically Baby
Website: http://weeshop.com
Customer Service: 888-254-8780
Bedding, baby care, clothing, and pregnancy.

Bassett
Website: http://www.bassettfurniture.com
Customer Service: 540-629-6000
Bedding/furniture.

Beautiful Baby
Website: http://www.bbaby.com
Customer Service: 903-295-2229
Bedding.

Bebe Chic
Website: http://www.bebechic.com
Customer Service: 201-447-6473 Fax: 201-447-1101
Bedding.

Bellini
Website: http://www.bellini.com
Customer Service: 800-332-BABY
Bedding/furniture.

Bob the Builder
Website: http://www.bobthebuilder.com
Customer Service: 888-427-0720
Bob the Builder everything - clothing, bedding, toys, etc.

Brandee Danielle
Website: http://www.brandeedanielle.com
Customer Service: 903-295-2229
Signature bedding.

Carter's
Website: http://www.carters.com
Customer Service: 888-782-9548
Bedding and clothing.

Celebrations
Website: http://www.baby-celebrations.com
Customer Service: 310-532-2499
Bedding.

Character Products
Website: http://www.characterproducts.com
Customer Service: online form
Popular character products. Clothing, bedding, baby care, feeding.

Cherish & Joy Kidstuff
Website: http://www.cherishandjoy.com
Customer Service: 888-745-5922
Baby gear, bedding, and clothing.

Cherished Moments
Website: http://www.cherishedmoments.com
Customer Service: 713-957-2764 Fax: 713-957-2764
Toys, bedding, parenting, baby names, and baby gear.

Child Craft Furniture
Website: http://www.childcraftind.com
Customer Service: 812-883-3111
Bedding/furniture.

Comfort Living
Website: http://www.baby-store.net
Customer Service: 877-378-4411
Feeding, health/safety, baby gear, bedding, toys, pregnancy.

Comfort Silkie
Website: http://www.comfortsilkie.com
Customer Service: 800-226-2229
Bedding.

Company Store, The
Website: http://www.thecompanystore.com
Customer Service: 800-323-8000
Toys, bedding, clothing, and baby care.

Cookie Baby Inc.
Website: http://www.cookiebabyinc.com
Customer Service: 877-787-0088
Personalized baby products., toys, bedding and gifts.

Custom Crib Sets by Audrey
Website: http://www.audrey-enterp.com
Customer Service: audrey.wood@juno.com
Bedding.

D.E.X. Products
Website: http://www.dexproducts.com
Customer Service: 800-546-1996
Bedding and baby gear.

Daisy Kingdom
Website: http://www.daisykingdom.com
Customer Service: 503-222-4281
Bedding.

Decorate Today
Website: http://www.decoratetoday.com
Customer Service: 800-735-5300
Baby room décor.

Dream On Me
Website: http://www.dreamonme.com
Customer Service: 877-768-5500 Fax: 718-832-8148
Bedding and accessories.

Dutalier
Website: http://www.dutalier.com
Customer Service: 800-363-9817
Rocking chairs and gliders.

E Baby Station
Website: http://ebabystation.com
Customer Service: 706-863-4452 Fax: 706-863-4452
Bedding, gifts, pregnancy, baby care, gear, clothing, and toys.

EStyle
Website: http://www.estyle.com
Customer Service: 877-ESTYLES
Bedding, toys, clothing, pregnancy, gifts, and baby gear.

Eco Baby
Website: http://www.ecobaby.com
Customer Service: 800-596-7450
Pregnancy, bedding, baby care, books/music, and clothing

Express Baby
Website: http://www.expressbaby.com
Customer Service: 800-600-0410
Baby care, gear, feeding, bedding, gifts, safety, and clothing.

Furniture Fan
Website: http://www.furniturefan.com
Customer Service: jonk@furniturefan.com
Furniture and accessories.

Fy Home
Website: http://www.fyhome.com
Customer Service: 888-242-7448 Fax: 763-757-1877
Baby room décor.

Garden Lane
Website: http://www.gardenlane.com
Customer Service: 888-388-7885
Baby care and bedding.

Gliders Direct
Website: http://www.glidersdirect.com
Customer Service: 800-672-6962
Rocking chairs and gliders.

Great Beginnings
Website: http://www.childrensfurniture.com
Customer Service: 800-886-7099
Bedding/furniture, baby gear, toys, safety, books/music, and gifts.

Happy Scraps
Website: http://www.happyscraps.com
Customer Service: 813-986-5767 Fax: 813-986-9585
Personalized baby room décor.

House of Hatten
Website: http://www.houseofhatten.com
Customer Service: 800-542-8836
Children's apparel and baby bedding.

Infantino
Website: http://www.infantino.com
Customer Service: 800-365-8182 Fax: 858-457-0181
Toys, bedding, and baby gear.

Kazmar
Website: http://www.kazmar.com
Customer Service: 888-834-PASH Fax: 530-821-0828
Pashmina baby blankets.

Kid Fancies
Website: http://www.kidfancies.com
Customer Service: 877-376-2992
Distinctive furnishings and gifts for children.

Kids II
Website: http://www.kidsii.com
Customer Service: 770-751-0442
Toys, bedding, baby care, and baby gear.

Kids Etc
Website: http://www.kids-etc.com
Customer Service: 949-495-5828
Bedding.

Kittrich
Website: http://www.kittrich.com
Customer Service: 800-497-2867
Baby room décor, wallpaper, paint, etc.

Lambs and Ivy
Website: http://www.lambsivy.com
Customer Service: 800-34-LAMBS
Bedding, gifts, and safety.

Lamby Nursery Collection
Website: http://www.lamby.com
Customer Service: 800-669-0527
Baby gear accessories and bedding.

Lane Kids Furniture
Website: http://www.lanekids.com
Customer Service: 800-750-LANE
Furniture.

Laura Ashley
Website: http://www.sumersault.com
Customer Service: 800-232-3006
Bedding.

Leachco 📖
Website: http://www.leachco.com
Customer Service: 800-525-1050
Bedding, baby care, health/safety, baby gear, and pregnancy.

Legacy Linens
Website: http://www.legacylinens.com
Customer Service: online form
Bedding.

Lexington
Website: http://www.lexington.com
Customer Service: 800-539-4636
Furniture.

Little Bobby Creations
Website: http://www.littlebobbycreations.com
Customer Service: 219-662-6368
Personalized gift cards and baby room décor.

Little Miss Liberty
Website: http://www.crib.com
Customer Service: 800-RND-CRIB
Bedding/furniture.

Luv n' Care
Website: http://www.luvncare.com
Customer Service: 888-LUVNCARE
Baby care, toys, and bedding.

Meijer Baby Club
Website: http://www.meijer.com/babyclub
Customer Service: 800-543-3704
Feeding, baby gear, bedding, baby care, pregnancy, and toys.

Million Dollar Baby
Website: http://www.milliondollarbaby.com
Customer Service: 323-728-8866
Bedding.

Morigeau/Lepine
Website: http://www.goodnightben.com.com
Customer Service: 800-326-2121
Bedding/furniture.

My Dog Spot
Website: http://www.mydogspot4kids.com
Customer Service: 858-259-7200 Fax: 858-259-7365
Bedding.

My Magnetic Creations
Website: http://www.mymagneticcreations.com
Customer Service: 800-850-0113
Magnetize your walls and decorate.

Neat Stuff Gifts
Website: http://www.neatstuffgifts.com
Customer Service: 800-586-9278 Fax: 732-846-9796
Gifts, toys, and bedding.

Noel Joanna, Inc. (NoJo)
Website: http://www.nojo.com
Customer Service: 800-854-8760
Safety, furniture, and bedding.

Nursery Bright
Website: http://www.nurserybright.com
Customer Service: 877-BABY-959
Baby care, furniture, bedding, safety, clothing, and gear.

Nursery Rhymes
Website: http://www.nurseryrhymes.com
Customer Service: 519-743-1321 Fax: 519-743-1681
Baby gear, furniture/bedding, toys, and safety.

Nursery Time
Website: http://www.nursery-time.com
Customer Service: 859-233-3148
Furniture and bedding.

Pali
Website: http://www.paliusa.com
Customer Service: 630-953-9519
Bedding/furniture.

Parent Hub
Website: http://www.parenthub.com
Customer Service: info@parenthub.com
Parenting, clothing, funiture, toys, and books.

Pine Creek Bedding
Website: http://www.pinecreekbedding.com
Customer Service: 800-218-7475
Bedding.

Poshtots
Website: http://www.poshtots.com
Customer Service: 866-POSH-TOTS Fax: 804-935-0844
Bedding and gifts.

Pottery Barn Kids 📖

Website: http://www.potterybarnkids.com
Customer Service: 888-779-5176 Fax: 702-363-2541
Bedding, furniture, and gifts.

Pregnant Inc.

Website: http://www.pregnantinc.com
Customer Service: 626-288-6220
Bedding, furniture, and baby gear.

Prince Lionheart

Website: http://www.princelionheart.com
Customer Service: 800-544-1132 Fax: 805-982-9442
Bedding, baby care, and safety.

Priss Prints

Website: http://www.prissprints.com
Customer Service: 800-323-5999
Baby room decor.

Quiltex

Website: http://www.quiltex.com
Customer Service: 800-237-3636
Bedding.

R R Gifts 📖

Website: http://www.rrgifts.com/thomas.html
Customer Service: 888-RRGIFTS
Toys, books, videos, bedding, clothing, and more.

Ragazzi

Website: http://www.ragazzi.com
Customer Service: 514-324-7886
Bedding.

Red Calliope

Website: http://www.redcalliope.com
Customer Service: 800-421-0526
Safety, bedding, maternity, and baby care.

Regal

Website: http://www.mvmills.com
Customer Service: 800-845-3251
Bedding.

Rocking Chairs
Website: http://www.rocking-chairs.com
Customer Service: 800-4-ROCKER
Furniture.

Royal Nursery, The
Website: http://www.newborngifts.com
Customer Service: 858-450-1317
Gifts, music, baby care, bedding, clothing, etc.

Royal Velvet
Website: http://www.royalvelvet.com
Customer Service: 800-476-7112
Baby care and bedding.

Rumble Tuff
Website: http://www.rumbletuff.com
Customer Service: 800-524-9607 Fax: 208-375-2511
Furniture.

Russ Berrie & Company
Website: http://www.russberrie.com
Customer Service: 800-358-8278
Plush toys, gifts and bedding accessories.

Selfix
Website: http://www.hpii.com
Customer Service: 800-327-3534
Closet organizers.

Sheep Skin Express
Website: http://www.sheepskinexpress.com
Customer Service: 866-287-8495 Fax: 877-890-7773
Sheep skin products such as rugs and car seat covers.

Simmons
Website: http://www.simmonsjp.com
Customer Service: 920-882-2140
Bedding/Furniture.

Storkcraft
Website: http://www.storkcraft.com
Customer Service: 604-275-4242 Fax: 604-274-9727
Furniture and safety.

Stork Delivers, The
Website: http://www.thestorkdelivers.com
Customer Service: 800-94-BABYS
Gift baskets, bedding, and announcements.

Sunsational Kids
Website: http://www.sunsationalkids.com
Customer Service: 910-353-6561 Fax: 910-353-5153
Toys, books, music, furniture, and clothing.

Sweet Pea Company
Website: http://www.sweetpeacompany.com
Customer Service: online form
Gifts, bedding, music, and parenting.

Target Lullaby Club
Website: http://www.target.com
Customer Service: 800-888-9333
Everything baby.

Toys R Us
Website: http://www.toysrus.com
Customer Service: 800-TOYS-R-Us
Toys, feeding, baby care, gear,bedding/furniture, books/music.

This Baby of Mine
Website: http://www.thisbabyofmine.com
Customer Service: 877-572-6427 Fax: 775-239-1944
Announcements, bedding, books, clothing, baby care, toys.

Triboro Quilt Manufacturing
Website: http://www.triboro.com
Customer Service: 800-227-2077
Bedding.

Tuttibella
Website: http://www.tuttibella.com
Customer Service: 877-279-9391
Bedding, furniture, clothes, toys, baby gear, and more.

USA Baby
Website: http://www.usababy.com
Customer Service: 800-323-4108
Furniture and bedding.

Vermont Precision
Website: http://www.vtprecision.com
Customer Service: 802-888-7974
Furniture.

Warm Fuzzys
Website: http://www.warmfuzzys.net/baby.htm
Customer Service: 419-824-7844
Personalized bedding, and announcements.

Yahoo
Website: http://shoppingyahoo.com
Customer Service: online form
Furniture, clothing, bedding, baby gear, and more.

Books, Music, Magazines, Videos, and Educational Entertainment

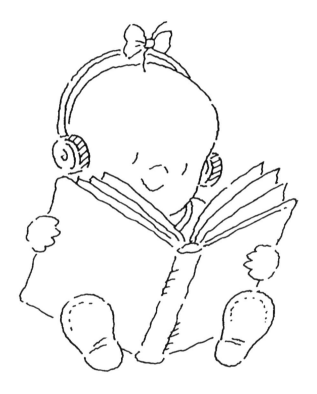

Able Baby
Website: http://www.ablebaby.com
Customer Service: ablebabyco@aol.com
Safety, baby care, bedding, books/music/videos, toys.

All Baby
Website: http://www.allbaby.com
Customer Service: 800-781-7171
Books, gifts, and names.

A Smart Baby
Website: http://www.asmartbaby.com
Customer Service: 877-310-6647
Toys, gifts, books/videos, and announcements.

Attachments
Website: http://www.attachmentscatalog.com
Customer Service: 800-873-5023
Toys, breastfeeding, gifts, books, and baby gear.

Audio Therapy
Website: http://www.babygotosleep.com
Customer Service: 800-537-7748
Help your baby stop crying and fussing with music.

Babies Classics
Website: http://www.babiesclassics.com
Customer Service: 888-454-BABY
Gift baskets, books/music, and clothing.

Babies-R-Us
Website: http://www.babiesrus.com
Customer Service: 800-BABYRUS
Everything baby.

Baby Abby
Website: http://www.babyabby.com
Customer Service: 800-972-7357 Fax: 303-777-6117
Baby care, clothing, pregnancy, baby gear, safety, gifts.

Baby and Family
Website: http://www.babyandfamily.com
Customer Service: 1-303-302-357 (Australia)
Infant videos.

Baby Box
Website: http://babybox.com
Customer Service: 800-373-8216
Boutique baby gifts, books/music, clothing, bedding, and toys.

Baby Bumblebee 📖
Website: http://www.babybumblebee.com
Customer Service: 888-984-5500
Educational videos and books.

Baby Bunz
Website: http://www.babybunz.com
Customer Service: 800-676-4559 Fax: 360-354-1203
Baby care, clothing, bedding, toys, books, feeding.

Baby College
Website: http://www.babycollege.com
Customer Service: 800-483-3383
Infant educational videos.

Baby Concepts
Website: http://www.babyconcepts.com
Customer Service: info@babyconcepts.com
Baby care, clothing, feeding, books, and gifts.

Baby Einstein
Website: http://www.babyeinstein.com
Customer Service: 800-793-1454
Educational videos, books, and more.

Genius Baby
Website: http://www.geniusbaby.com
Customer Service: 704-573-4500 Fax: 704-545-5716
Baby gifts, books and toys.

Baby Go To Sleep
Website: http://www.babygotosleep.com
Customer Service: 800-537-7748
Help your baby stop crying and fussing with music.

Baby Land
Website: http://www.babyland.com
Customer Service: stork@babyland.com
Announcements, books, and parenting.

Baby Land / Baby Land Kids Room
Website: http://www.babyland-kidsroom.com
Customer Service: 888-316-8952
Bedding, baby gear, feeding, safety, and gifts.

Baby Massage
Website: http://www.babymassage.net
Customer Service: 877-782-6476 Fax: 775-855-5215
Baby massage videos.

Baby Navigator
Website: http://www.babynavigator.com
Customer Service: online form
Safety, bedding, feeding, toys, baby care, clothing, gear, books.

Baby Net Center
Website: http://www.babynetcenter.com
Customer Service: online form
Clothing, bedding, feeding, baby gear, baby care, books, gifts.

Baby Outlet
Website: http://www.babyoutlet.com
Customer Service: home@babyoutlet.com
Books/music and baby names.

Baby Resource
Website: http://www.babyresource.com
Customer Service: online form
Toys, health/safety, and books/music.

Baby Scapes
Website: http://www.babyscapes.com
Customer Service: 888-441-KIDS
Parenting and books/music.

Baby Science
Website: http://www.babyscience.com
Customer Service: pageone@kawartha.com
Books and music.

Baby Shop Magazine
Website: http://www.babyshopmagazine.com
Customer Service: 412-531-942 Fax: 412-531-2004
Magazine.

Baby Shower
Website: http://www.baby-shower.com
Customer Service: online form
Announcements, parenting, books/music, and gifts.

Baby Signs
Website: http://www.babysigns.com
Customer Service: 800-995-0226
Parenting and books/music.

Baby Songs
Website: http://www.babysongs.com
Customer Service: 323-653-4431 Fax: 323-801-2108
Music.

Baby Talk
Website: http://www.babytalk.com
Customer Service: online form
Parenting magazine.

Baby Tunes
Website: http://www.babytunes.com
Customer Service: popi@babytunes.com
Music.

Baby Universe
Website: http://www.babyuniverse.com
Customer Service: 877-615-BABY Fax: 954-523-9881
Safety, feeding, books/music, baby care, gear, toys, bedding.

Babynet Center
Website: http://www.babynetcenter.com
Customer Service: online form
Books/music, clothing, feeding, bedding, toys, baby gear.

Barney for Baby
Website: http://www.barneyforbaby.com
Customer Service: 800-418-2371
Barney clothing, boons, music, toys, gifts, etc.

Bebe Sounds
Website: http://www.bebesounds.com
Customer Service: 800-233-1196 Fax: 212-736-6762
Baby gear and music.

Big Kids Video
Website: http://www.bigkidsvideo.com
Customer Service: 800-477-7811
Children's videos.

Bizzy Bum
Website: http://www.bizzybum.com
Customer Service: 888-243-2977
Books and music.

Birth and Baby
Website: http://www.birthandbaby.com
Customer Service: 888-398-7987
Books/music, pregnancy, and clothing.

Bob the Builder
Website: http://www.bobthebuilder.com
Customer Service: 888-427-0720
Bob the Builder everything -clothing, bedding, toys, books, etc.

Book Adventure
Website: http://www.bookadventure.com
Customer Service: 410-843-8000
Books.

Build Your Baby's Brain
Website: http://www.buildyourbabysbrain.com
Customer Service: 800-255-7514
Build your baby's brain through the power of music.

C. R. Gibson
Website: http://www.crgibson.com
Customer Service: 800-541-8880 Fax: 615-902-2298
Photo and memory books for baby.

Character Products
Website: http://www.characterproducts.com
Customer Service: online form
Popular character products - clothing, bedding, baby care, books.

Child Birth Class
Website: http://www.childbirthclass.com
Customer Service: 909-985-6151
Child birth classes and videos.

Children's Book of the Month Club
Website: http://www.cbomc.com
Customer Service: customerservice@cbomc.com
Children's books.

Christian Expression
Website: http://www.christianexpression.com
Customer Service: 401-942-3929 Fax: 401-944-0913
Personalized products, books/music, and gifts.

Creative Memories
Website: http://www.creativememories.com
Customer Service: online form
Scrapbooking.

Disney Learning
Website: http://www.disneylearning.org
Customer Service: 800-688-1520
Interactive games on line.

Dragon Fly Toys
Website: http://www.dragonflytoys.com
Customer Service: 800-308-2208 Fax: 204-453-2320
Toys and books.

E Guide Baby
Website: http://www.eguidebaby.com
Customer Service: 713-721-5256
Books, music, videos, and software.

E News
Website: http://www.enews.com/riskfree
Customer Service: 800-932-9595
Order magazines online.

E Pregnancy
Website: http://www.epregnancy.com
Customer Service: 925-447-6667 Fax: 925-937-7203
Pregnancy, books, and baby names.

Earth Baby
Website: http://www.earthbaby.com
Customer Service: 877-602-6800
Books/music, clothing, and baby care.

Eco Baby 📖
Website: http://www.ecobaby.com
Customer Service: 800-596-7450
Pregnancy, bedding, baby care, books/music, and clothing

Education
Website: http://www.education.com
Customer Service: 800-545-7677
Parenting and books.

Educating Baby
Website: http://www.educatingbaby.com
Customer Service: 800-533-5392
Parenting and books.

Family Home Entertainment
Website: http://www.familyhomeent.com
Customer Service: 310-255-3942 Fax: 310-255-3990
Large selection of movies and fun for the family.

Family Life Magazine
Website: http://www.familylifemag.com
Customer Service: 800-682-7667
Parenting and magazines.

Family On Board 📖
Website: http://www.familyonboard.com
Customer Service: 800-793-2075 Fax: 603-588-3177
Coloring books and games for traveling.

First Toys
Website: http://www.firsttoys.com
Customer Service: 800-210-7318
Toys, books, and music.

For Babies
Website: http://www.4babies.com
Customer Service: 510-768-1444
Books, parenting, clothing, and baby names.

Gentle Mom
Website: http://www.gentlemom.com
Customer Service: 877-833-BABY
Baby gear, baby care, books/music, and parenting.

Golden Books
Website: http://www.goldenbooks.com
Customer Service: 212-547-6700
Children's books.

Great American Audio
Website: http://www.greatamericanaudio.com
Customer Service: 800-675-2834
Lullaby music and books.

Great Beginnings
Website: http://www.childrensfurniture.com
Customer Service: 800-886-7099
Bedding/furniture, baby gear, toys, safety, books/music, and gifts.

Imaginarium
Website: http://www.imaginarium.com
Customer Service: 88-TOYOLOGY
Toys, books, and music.

Infant Learning
Website: http://www.infantlearning.com
Customer Service: 888-732-3888
Educational videos.

Kidology Toys
Website: http://www.kidologytoys.com
Customer Service: 800-995-4436 Fax: 800-995-0506
Educational toys.

Klutz
Website: http://www.klutz.com
Customer Service: 800-737-4123
Books and toys

Leap Frog
Website: http://www.leapfrog.com
Customer Service: 800-701-LEAP
Books and educational toys.

Learning Co.
Website: http://www.learningco.com
Customer Service: 800-543-9778
Educational software for children 0 - 3 and up.

Lullabies From Home
Website: http://anitakruse.com/main.htm
Customer Service: akk@nol.net
Lullaby music.

Lullaby Shoppe
Website: http://www.lullabyshoppe.com
Customer Service: 509-935-8809
Gift baskets and lullaby music.

M H Kids
Website: http://www.mhkids.com
Customer Service: 800-305-5571
Books.

M V O Records
Website: http://www.mvorecords.com
Customer Service: 206-567-4831
Music.

Mom's Love, A
Website: http://www.amomslove.com
Customer Service: online form
Parenting, magazine.

Mommy Magic
Website: http://www.mommymagic.com
Customer Service: thestaff@mommymagic.com
Books, music, gifts.

Mother and Baby
Website: http://www.motherandbaby.co.uk
Customer Service: UK
Mother and Baby Magazine.

Music For Little People
Website: http://www.mflp.com
Customer Service: 800-346-4445
Music and videos.

Museum Tour
Website: http://www.museumtour.com
Customer Service: 800-360-9116
Books, music, games, puzzles and creative play.

MVP Home Entertainment
Website: http://www.mvphomevideo.com
Customer Service: 800-772-6847
Young children's videos.

My Baby Connection
Website: http://www.mybabyconnection.com
Customer Service: webmaster@mybabyconnection.com
Announcements, clothing, gifts, books, and much more.

Natural Mom
Website: http://www.naturalmom.com
Customer Service: 608-242-0200
Health, pregnancy, books, and bath care.

Nick Jr.
Website: http://www.nickjr.com
Customer Service: Online form
Games, toys, books, videos, etc.

Nickelodeon
Website: http://www.nick.com
Customer Service: Online form
Games, toys, books, videos, etc.

Nickelodeon
Website: http://www.nickelodeon.com
Customer Service: Online form
Games, toys, books, videos, etc.

Parent Hub
Website: http://www.parenthub.com
Customer Service: info@parenthub.com
Parenting, clothing, funiture, toys, and books.

Parenting
Website: http://www.parenting.com
Customer Service: online fom
Parenting magazine.

Paenting Concepts
Website: http://www.parentingconcepts.com
Customer Service: 800-727-3683
Baby gear, books /music, parenting, toys, and gifts.

Perfectly Safe 📖
Website: http://www.perfectlysafe.com
Customer Service: 800-837-5437
Safety and books.

Pitter Patter Productions
Website: http://www.pitterpatterproductions.com
Customer Service: 503-598-9861 Fax: 503-213-6217
Music.

Popular Baby Names
Website: http://www.popularbabynames.com
Customer Service: online form
Baby names, books, and music.

Preemie Store and More, The 📖
Website: http://www.preemie.com
Customer Service: 800-755-4852
Preemie clothing.

Pregnancy Weekly
Website: http://www.pregnancyweekly.com
Customer Service: online form
Pregnancy and baby names magazine.

PTA
Website: http://www.pta.org
Customer Service: 800-307-4PTA Fax: 312-670-6783
Parenting magazine.

R R Gifts 📖
Website: http://www.rrgifts.com/thomas.html
Customer Service: 888-RRGIFTS
Toys, books, videos, bedding, clothing, and more.

Random House
Website: http://www.randomhouse.com/kids
Customer Service: 800-800-3246 Fax: 212-940-7381
Books.

Right Start, The 📖
Website: http://www.therightstart.com
Customer Service: 800-LITTLE-1
Books, baby gear, health, safety, and much more.

Rock Me Baby Records
Website: http://www.rockmebabyrecords.com
Customer Service: 415-255-4719
Music.

Royal Nursery, The
Website: http://www.newborngifts.com
Customer Service: 858-450-1317
Gifts, music, baby care, bedding, clothing, books.

Scholastic
Website: http://www.scholastic.com
Customer Service: online form
Parenting and books.

Sensory Resources
Website: http://www.sensoryresources.com
Customer Service: 888-357-5867 Fax: 702-891-9988
Books, videos, and audio tapes.

Sesame Street
Website: http://www.sesamestreet.com
Customer Service: online form
Games, parenting, music, pregnancy, etc.

Sesame Street Workshop
Website: http://www.sesameworkshop.org
Customer Service: online form
Stories, games, parenting, music, pregnancy, etc

Sign to Me
Website: http://www.sign2me.com
Customer Service: 206-361-0307 Fax: 206-362-2025
Communicate with your baby through sign language.

Sleep Baby
Website: http://www.sleepbaby.com
Customer Service: 888-795-0555
Parenting, videos.

Slumber Sounds
Website: http://www.slumbersounds.com
Customer Service: 425-823-2010
Music to help your baby fall asleep.

Smarter Kids Software 📖
Website: http://www.smarterkidssoftware.com
Customer Service: 888-881-6001
Educational software.

Someday Baby Lullabyes
Website: http://www.lullabyes.com
Customer Service: 800-965-BABY
Lullaby music.

Sony Wonder
Website: http://www.sonywonder.com
Customer Service: online form
Children's music.

Sunsational Kids
Website: http://www.sunsationalkids.com
Customer Service: 910-353-6561 Fax: 910-353-5153
Toys, books, music, furniture, and clothing.

Super Baby Food
Website: http://www.superbabyfood.com
Customer Service: 866-BABY-BOOK
Baby food book.

Sweet Pea Company
Website: http://www.sweetpeacompany.com
Customer Service: online form
Gifts, bedding, music, and parenting.

Target Lullaby Club
Website: http://www.target.com
Customer Service: 800-888-9333
Everything baby.

Tangerine Bear
Website: http://www.tangerinebear.com
Customer Service: online form
Videos and toys.

That's Another Story
Website: http://www.thatsanotherstory.com
Customer Service: online form
Books.

This Baby of Mine
Website: http://www.thisbabyofmine.com
Customer Service: 877-572-6427 Fax: 775-239-1944
Announcements, bedding, books, clothing, care, toys.

Tiny Love
Website: http://www.tinylove.com
Customer Service: 888-TINY-LOVE
Soft developmental toys and magazine.

Tivola Publishing
Website: http://www.tivola.com
Customer Service: 212-431-4420 Fax: 212-431-4537
Books.

Toys R Us
Website: http://www.toysrus.com
Customer Service: 800-TOYS-R-Us
Toys, feeding, baby care, gear,bedding/furniture, books/music.

True Blue Music
Website: http://www.bigkidsvideo.com
Customer Service: 800-477-8711
Music, video, and software.

W J Fantasy Publishing
Website: http://www.wjfantasy
Customer Service: 800-222-7529
Books and toys.

Zany Brainy
Website: http://www.zanybrainy.com
Customer Service: 877-WOW-KIDS
Developmental toys and books.

Clothing

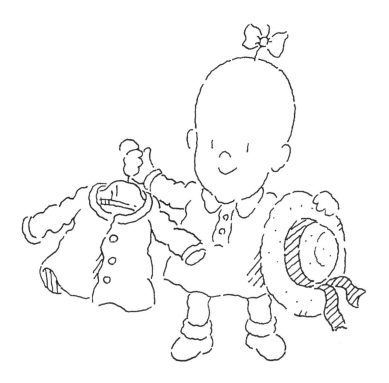

Adorable Baby Gifts
Website: http://www.adorablebabygifts.com
Customer Service: 713-666-0844
Gifts, clothing, and baby names.

ADZ Baby Gifts
Website: http://www.adz-baby-gifts.com
Customer Service: 800-464-0042
Clothing, toys, and gift baskets.

Alexis
Website: http://www.alexisusa.com
Customer Service: 800-253-9476
Clothing.

Alternative Baby
Website: http://www.alternativebaby.com
Customer Service: 800-469-1126
Baby care, gear, clothing, pregnancy, toys, and gifts baskets.

American Baby Company
Website: http://www.americanbaby.com
Customer Service: 909-597-9070
Clothing, toys, pregnancy, parenting, and gifts.

Annacris
Website: http://www.annacris.com
Customer Service: 800-281-ANNA
Maternity clothing.

Babblin' Babies
Website: http://www.babblinbabies.com
Customer Service: 800-217-8141
Clothing.

Babies Classics
Website: http://www.babiesclassics.com
Customer Service: 888-454-BABY
Gift baskets, books/music, and clothing.

Babies-R-Us
Website: http://www.babiesrus.com
Customer Service: 800-BABYRUS
Everything baby- Baby Superstore.

Baby Abby
Website: http://www.babyabby.com
Customer Service: 800-972-7357 Fax: 303-777-6117
Baby care, gear, clothing, pregnancy, safety, gifts.

Baby Ant
Website: http://www.babyant.com
Customer Service: online form
Toys, clothing, health, bedding, and gifts.

Baby Bargains
Website: http://www.babybargains.com
Customer Service: 540-899-6090
Toys, pregnancy, and clothing.

Baby Bazaar
Website: http://www.babybazaar.com
Customer Service: 877-543-7186
Clothing, baby gear, toys, bedding, and gifts.

Baby Becoming 📖
Website: http://www.babybecoming.com
Customer Service: 888-666-6910
Maternity and nursing clothing.

Baby Bee Hats
Website: http://www.babybeehats.com
Customer Service: info@babybeehats.com
Baby hats.

Baby Bloomers
Website: http://www.babyblooms.com
Customer Service: 521-633-2642
Clothing and gifts.

Baby Boom
Website: http://www.babyboom1.com
Customer Service: 800-929-4666
Gifts, pregnancy, clothing, and toys.

Baby Box
Website: http://babybox.com
Customer Service: 800-373-8216
Boutique baby gifts, books/music, clothing, bedding, and toys.

Baby Bunz
Website: http://www.babybunz.com
Customer Service: 800-676-4559 Fax: 360-354-1203
Baby care, clothing, bedding, toys, books, feeding.

Baby Catalogue, The 📖
Website: http://www.thebabycatalogue.com
Customer Service: London
Clothing, feeding, baby care, gear, bedding, safety, and toys.

Baby Concepts
Website: http://www.babyconcepts.com
Customer Service: info@babyconcepts.com
Baby care, clothing, feeding, books, and gifts.

Baby Corner, The
Website: http://www.thebabycorner.com
Customer Service: 812-867-3759
Baby care, gear, pregnancy, parenting, clothing, toys, bedding.

Baby Gap
Website: http://www.babygap.com
Customer Service: 800-427-7895
Clothing.

Baby Guess
Website: http://www.babyguess.com
Customer Service: 877-44-GUESS
Clothing.

Baby Heirlooms
Website: http://www.babyheirlooms.com
Customer Service: 800-340-8838
Toys, clothing, and gifts.

Baby Mountain
Website: http://www.babymountain.com
Customer Service: mail@babymountain.com
Announcements, clothing, feeding, names, toys, safety, bedding.

Baby n' Mom
Website: http://www.baby-n-mom.com
Customer Service: webmaster@best-toys-prices.com
Clothing, bedding, parenting, names, and baby gear.

Baby Navigator
Website: http://www.babynavigator.com
Customer Service: online form
Safety, bedding, feeding, toys, baby care, gear, clothing, books.

Baby Net Center
Website: http://www.babynetcenter.com
Customer Service: online form
Clothing, bedding, feeding, baby gear, baby care, books, gifts.

Baby Style
Website: http://www.babystyle.com
Customer Service: 877-ESTYLES
Bedding, toys, clothing, baby gear, baby care.

Baby Supermall
Website: http://www.babysupermall.com
Customer Service: online form
Baby care, feeding, toys, bedding, clothing, health/safety.

Baby T's
Website: http://www.babyts.com
Customer Service: 800-3BABYTs Fax: 530-885-0726
Clothing and gifts.

Baby Tees
Website: http://www.babytees.com
Customer Service: online form
Humorous baby wear.

Baby Ultimate
Website: http://www.babyultimate.com
Customer Service: 877-724-4537
Clothing and toys.

Baby Universe
Website: http://www.babyuniverse.com
Customer Service: 877-615-BABY Fax: 954-523-9881
Safety, feeding, books/music, baby care, gear, toys, bedding.

Babyking
Website: http://babyking.com
Customer Service: 800-424-BABY
Toys, feeding, clothing, baby care, and gifts.

Babynet Center
Website: http://www.babynetcenter.com
Customer Service: online form
Books/music, clothing, feeding, bedding, toys, baby gear.

Babyworks
Website: http://www.babyworks.com
Customer Service: 800-422-2910
Feeding, toys, babycare, bedding, clothing.

Barney for Baby
Website: http://www.barneyforbaby.com
Customer Service: 800-418-2371
Barney clothing, books, music, toys, gifts, etc.

Bareware
Website: http://bareware.net
Customer Service: 877-9 DIAPER
Clothing, toys, baby care, gear, and pregnancy.

Basic Comfort
Website: http://www.basiccomfort.com
Customer Service: 800-456-8687
Bedding, clothing, baby care, and health/safety.

Basically Baby
Website: http://weeshop.com
Customer Service: 888-254-8780
Bedding, baby care, clothing, and pregnancy.

Bio Bottoms 📖
Website: http://www.biobottoms.com
Customer Service: 800-766-1254
Clothing.

Birth and Baby
Website: http://www.birthandbaby.com
Customer Service: 888-398-7987
Books/music, pregnancy, and clothing.

Bloom N' Fashion
Website: http://www.bloom-n.com
Customer Service: online form
Maternity clothing.

Bob the Builder
Website: http://www.bobthebuilder.com
Customer Service: 888-427-0720
Bob the Builder everything - clothing, bedding, toys, books, etc.

Bobux USA
Website: http://www.bobuxusa.com
Customer Service: 800-315-3039 Fax: 303-663-2594
Baby shoes.

Boys Enb
Website: http://www.boysenb.com
Customer Service: 802-767-6064
Clothing.

Burlington Coat Factory
Website: http://www.coat.com
Customer Service: online form
Discount clothing.

Canada Baby Works
Website: http://www.canadababyworks.com
Customer Service: 877-531-BABY
Clothing, baby care, gear, toys, and pregnancy.

Carter's
Website: http://www.carters.com
Customer Service: 888-782-9548
Bedding and clothing.

Character Products
Website: http://www.characterproducts.com
Customer Service: online form
Popular character products - clothing, bedding, baby care, feeding.

Cherish & Joy Kidstuff
Website: http://www.cherishandjoy.com
Customer Service: 888-745-5922
Baby gear, bedding, and clothing.

Children's Orchard
Website: http://www.childorch.com
Customer Service: 800-999-KIDS
Baby gear, toys, and clothing.

Children's Place
Website: http://www.childrensplace.com
Customer Service: 877-PLACEUSA
Clothing.

Company Store, The
Website: http://www.thecompanystore.com
Customer Service: 800-323-8000
Toys, bedding, clothing, and baby care.

Cuscraft
Website: http://www.cuscraft.com
Customer Service: 888-533-BABY
Birth announcements and clothing.

Dax & Coe
Website: http://www.daxandcoe.com
Customer Service: 415-356-2277
Maternity clothing.

E Baby Station
Website: http://ebabystation.com
Customer Service: 706-863-4452 Fax: 706-863-4452
Bedding, gifts, pregnancy, baby care, gear, clothing, and toys.

EStyle
Website: http://www.estyle.com
Customer Service: 877-ESTYLES
Bedding, toys, clothing, pregnancy, gifts, and baby gear.

Earth Baby
Website: http://www.earthbaby.com
Customer Service: 877-602-6800
Books/music, clothing, and baby care.

Eco Baby
Website: http://www.ecobaby.com
Customer Service: 800-596-7450
Pregnancy, bedding, baby care, books/music, and clothing

Eddie Bauer
Website: http://www.eddiebauer.com
Customer Service: 800-426-8020
Baby gear and clothing.

Euro Kids Clothes
Website: http://www.eurokidsclothes.com
Customer Service: 281-531-5331
Clothing.

Express Baby
Website: http://www.expressbaby.com
Customer Service: 800-600-0410
Baby care, gear, feeding, bedding, gifts, safety, and clothing.

Finetica Child
Website: http://www.fineticachild.com
Customer Service: 973-543-0053
Fine children's clothing.

Flap Happy
Website: http://www.flaphappy.com
Customer Service: 800-234-3527
Hats designed to protect children from the sun and bathing suits.

Flapdoodles
Website: http://www.flapdoodles.com
Customer Service: 302-731-9793
Upscale clothing.

For Babies
Website: http://www.4babies.com
Customer Service: 510-768-1444
Books, parenting, clothing, and baby names.

Garanimals
Website: http://www.garanimals.com
Customer Service: 800-759-4219
Affordable clothing.

Gerber Children's Wear
Website: http://www.gerberchildrenswear.com
Customer Service: 800-4-GERBER
Clothing.

Gifts for Baby
Website: http://www.giftsforbaby.com
Customer Service: 201-493-8722
Clothing, toys, and gifts.

Good Lad
Website: http://www.goodlad.com
Customer Service: 215-739-0200
Clothing.

Guess Baby
Website: http://www.guess.com/baby.asp
Customer Service: 877-44-GUESS
Clothing.

Gymboree
Website: http://www.gymboree.com
Customer Service: 800-520-PLAY
Clothing.

Hanna Andersson
Website: http://www.hannaandersson.com
Customer Service: 800-222-0544
Upscale clothing.

Health-Tex
Website: http://www.healthtex.com
Customer Service: 800-772-8336
Clothing.

Hi Baby
Website: http://www.hibaby.com
Customer Service: 888-HIBABY9
Preemie website, clothing, and baby contests.

House of Hatten
Website: http://www.houseofhatten.com
Customer Service: 800-542-8836
Upscale children's apparel and baby bedding.

Jake and Me
Website: http://www.jakeandme.com
Customer Service: 970-352-8802
Maternity, nursing, infant, and toddler clothing.

Keds
Website: http://www.keds.com
Customer Service: 800-270-6575
Shoes.

Kelly's Kids 📖
Website: http://www.kellyskids.com
Customer Service: 800-837-2066
Clothing, monogramming available.

Kidalog
Website: http://www.kidalog.com
Customer Service: 780-672-1763 Fax: 780-672-6942
Clothing, safety, breast pumps, and much more.

Kids R Us
Website: http://www.kidsrus.com
Customer Service: 800-869-7787
Clothing.

Kids Window, The
Website: http://www.thekidswindow.com
Customer Service: 877-504-3395
Clothing.

Lands End 📖
Website: http://www.landsend.com
Customer Service: 800-963-4816 Fax: 800-332-0103
Clothing.

Little Lids
Website: http://www.littlelids.com
Customer Service: info@littlelids.com
Hats.

Little Me
Website: http://www.littleme.com
Customer Service: 800-533-KIDS
Clothing - preemie clothing available.

Little Things Mean A Lot
Website: http://www.littlethingsmeanalot.com
Customer Service: 800-333-6036
Gifts and special occasion clothing.

L L Bean 📖
Website: http://www.llbean.com
Customer Service: 800-552-1968
Clothing.

Lollipops
Website: http://www.lollipopskidstuff.com
Customer Service: 859-266-2822
Boutique clothing.

Long Jacks
Website: http://www.longjacks.com
Customer Service: 977-LONG-JAC
Clothing.

Mom Shop
Website: http://www.momshop.com
Customer Service: 800-854-1213
Clothing, maternity, pregnancy, parenting.

Motherhood Maternity 📖
Website: http://www.motherhood.com
Customer Service: 800-4-MOM-2-BE
Maternity /nursing wear and baby names.

My Baby Connection
Website: http://www.mybabyconnection.com
Customer Service: webmaster@mybabyconnection.com
Announcements, clothing, gifts, books, and much more.

My Baby Shops
Website: http://www.mybabyshops.com
Customer Service: dawn@mybabyshops.com
Announcements, clothing, gifts, food, and much more.

Nest Mom
Website: http://www.nestmom.com
Customer Service: 301-824-6378
Baby gear, care, and clothing.

Nursery Bright
Website: http://www.nurserybright.com
Customer Service: 877-BABY-959
Baby care, furniture, bedding, safety, clothing and gear.

Oilily
Website: http://www.oililyusa.com
Customer Service: 800-977-7736
Upscale clothing.

Oink Baby
Website: http://www.oinkbaby.com
Customer Service: 866-592-0196
Clothing.

Old Navy
Website: http://www.oldnavy.com
Customer Service: 800-OLD-NAVY
Clothing and maternity.

One Hot Mama
Website: http://www.one hotmama.com
Customer Service: 800-217-3750
Clothing, nursing, baby gear.

One Step Ahead
Website: http://www.onestepahead.com
Customer Service: 800-274-8440
Clothing, baby care, gear, safety, pregnancy, and more.

Onesies
Website: http://www.1zies.com
Customer Service: 435-632-4123
Clothing.

Osh Kosh B'gosh
Website: http://www.oshkoshbgosh.com
Customer Service: 800-282-4674
Clothing.

Padders
Website: http://www.padders.com
Customer Service: 800-476-8312
Shoes.

Pampering Boutique
Website: http://www.pamperingboutique.com
Customer Service: 765-449-8514 Fax: same
Baby care, gifts, and clothing.

Parent Hub
Website: http://www.parenthub.com
Customer Service: info@parenthub.com
Parenting, clothing, funiture, toys, and books.

Patsy Aiken
Website: http://www.patsyaiken.com
Customer Service: 919-872-8789
Clothing.

Payless Shoes
Website: http://www.payless.com
Customer Service: 877-474-6379
Shoes.

Pea in the Pod, A
Website: http://www.apeainthepod.com
Customer Service: 877-273-2763
Maternity clothing.

Peaches 'n Cream
Website: http://www.peacheschildrenswear.com
Customer Service: online form
Upscale clothing.

Platypaws
Website: http://www.platypaws.com
Customer Service: 877-752-8979
Shoes.

Preemie Store and More, The 📖
Website: http://www.preemie.com
Customer Service: 800-755-4852
Preemie clothing.

Pump In Style
Website: http://www.pumpinstyle.com
Customer Service: 877-9-DIAPER Fax: 250-336-8848
Nursing, maternity, baby care, toys, clothing, etc.

R R Gifts 📖
Website: http://www.rrgifts.com/thomas.html
Customer Service: 888-RRGIFTS
Toys, books, videos, bedding, clothing, and more.

Ragsland
Website: http://www.ragsland.com
Customer Service: 800-242-0707 Fax: 225-926-3703
Upscale clothing.

Ritzy Rascals
Website: http://ritzyrascals.com
Customer Service: 866-URASCAL
Clothing and gifts.

Robeez
Website: http://www.robeez.com
Customer Service: 800-929-2623
Shoes.

Royal Baby
Website: http://www.royalbaby.com
Customer Service: 866-855-1945 Fax: 309-416-4472
Parenting, pregnancy, clothing, toys, gifts, etc.

Royal Nursery, The
Website: http://www.newborngifts.com
Customer Service: 858-450-1317
Gifts, music, baby care, bedding, clothing, books.

Sunsational Kids
Website: http://www.sunsationalkids.com
Customer Service: 910-353-6561 Fax: 910-353-5153
Toys, books, music, furniture, and clothing.

Talbot's Kids
Website: http://www.talbots.com
Customer Service: 800-543-7123
Clothing.

Target Lullaby Club
Website: http://www.target.com
Customer Service: 800-888-9333
Everything baby.

Tender Toes
Website: http://www.tendertoes.com
Customer Service: 800-666-LUNA
Shoes.

This Baby of Mine
Website: http://www.thisbabyofmine.com
Customer Service: 877-572-6427 Fax: 775-239-1944
Announcements, bedding, books, clothing, baby care, toys.

Toys R Us
Website: http://www.toysrus.com
Customer Service: 800-TOYS-R-Us
Toys, feeding, baby care, gear,bedding/furniture, books/music.

Tuttibella
Website: http://www.tuttibella.com
Customer Service: 877-279-9391
Bedding, furniture, clothes, toys, baby gear, and more.

Urban Baby
Website: http://www.urbanbaby.com
Customer Service: online form
Clothing and toys.

Wears the Baby
Website: http://www.wearsthebaby.com
Customer Service: 800-527-8985
Baby shoes.

Web Clothes
Website: http://www.wbclothes.com
Customer Service: 888-575-9303
Clothing.

Wes and Willy
Website: http://www.wesandwilly.com
Customer Service: online form
Clothing.

Warm Fuzzys
Website: http://www.warmfuzzys.net/baby.htm
Customer Service: 419-824-7844
Personalized bedding, and announcements.

Yahoo
Website: http://shoppingyahoo.com
Customer Service: online form
Furniture, clothing, bedding, baby gear, and more.

Zutano
Website: http://www.zutano.com
Customer Service: 800-287-5139
Clothing.

Gifts and Gifts Baskets

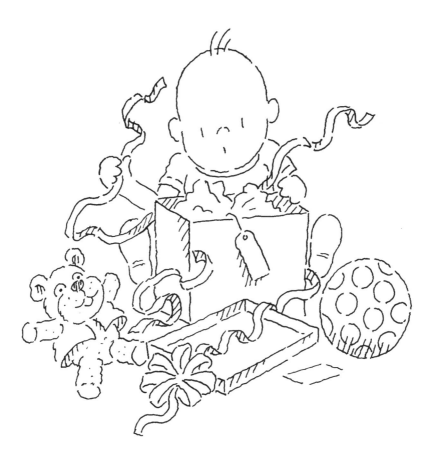

ABC Bronze
Website: http://www.abcbronze.com
Customer Service: 800-423-5678
Baby shoe bronzing.

Adorable Baby Gifts
Website: http://www.adorablebabygifts.com
Customer Service: 713-666-0844
Gifts, clothing, and baby names.

ADZ Baby Gifts
Website: http://www.adz-baby-gifts.com
Customer Service: 800-464-0042
Clothing, toys, and gift baskets.

Alternative Baby
Website: http://www.alternativebaby.com
Customer Service: 800-469-1126
Baby care, gear, clothing, pregnancy, toys, and gifts baskets.

American Baby Company
Website: http://www.americanbaby.com
Customer Service: 909-597-9070
Clothing, toys, pregnancy, parenting, and gifts.

American Bronzing Co
Website: http://www.abcbronze.com
Customer Service: 614-252-7388
Baby shoe bronzing.

Arrivals Baby Gifts
Website: http://www.arrivalsbabygifts.com
Customer Service: 800-741-0254
Toys, gifts, and bedding.

A Smart Baby
Website: http://www.asmartbaby.com
Customer Service: 877-310-6647
Toys, gifts, books/videos, and announcements.

Attachments 📖
Website: http://www.attachmentscatalog.com
Customer Service: 800-873-5023
Toys, breastfeeding, gifts, books, and baby gear.

BB Treasures
Website: http://www.bbtreasures.com
Customer Service: 866-966-BABY
Unique baby gifts.

Babies Classics
Website: http://www.babiesclassics.com
Customer Service: 888-454-BABY
Gift baskets, books/music, and clothing.

Babies-R-Us
Website: http://www.babiesrus.com
Customer Service: 800-BABYRUS
Everything baby.

Baby Ant
Website: http://www.babyant.com
Customer Service: online form
Toys, clothing, health, bedding, and gifts.

Baby Bazaar
Website: http://www.babybazaar.com
Customer Service: 877-543-7186
Clothing, baby gear, toys, bedding, and gifts.

Baby Bloomers
Website: http://www.babyblooms.com
Customer Service: 521-633-2642
Clothing and gifts.

Baby Boom
Website: http://www.babyboom1.com
Customer Service: 800-929-4666
Gifts, pregnancy, clothing and toys.

Baby Box
Website: http://babybox.com
Customer Service: 800-373-8216
Boutique baby gifts, books/music, clothing, bedding, and toys.

Baby Bundles of Joy
Website: http://www.babybundlesofjoy.com
Customer Service: 615-851-9730 Fax: 615-855-0759
Gift baskets.

Baby Cakes
Website: http://www.baby-cakes.com
Customer Service: 303-657-0799
Gifts for new parents and baby.

Baby Care
Website: http://babycare-sa.com
Customer Service: 866-343-2836
Baby gear, bedding, gifts, nursing, toys, and more.

Baby Concepts
Website: http://www.babyconcepts.com
Customer Service: info@babyconcepts.com
Baby care, clothing, feeding, books, and gifts.

Baby Corner, The
Website: http://www.thebabycorner.com
Customer Service: 812-867-3759
Baby care, gear, pregnancy, parenting, clothing, toys, bedding.

Baby Estore
Website: http://www.babyestore.com
Customer Service: 866-580-BABY
Breastfeeding supplies, bedding, and gifts.

Baby Gap
Website: http://www.babygap.com
Customer Service: 800-427-7895
Clothing for baby, children, and expectant mothers.

Baby Gift Idea
Website: http://www.babygiftidea.com
Customer Service: 904-880-2836
Gifts and nursery décor.

Baby Gift Place
Website: http://www.babygiftplace.com
Customer Service: 800-333-5690
Toys and gifts.

Baby Gifts 4 Less
Website: http://www.babygifts-4less.com
Customer Service: 877-378-4411
Baby gear, safety, bedding, toys, feeding, pregnancy, and gifts.

Baby Gifts by Ella
Website: http://www.babygiftsbyella.com
Customer Service: ella@babygiftsbyella.com
Original art and birth records.

Baby Gifts to Remember
Website: http://www.babygifts-to-remember.com
Customer Service: 800-353-2229 Fax: 800-433-9796
Personalized picture frames.

Baby Goodies
Website: http://www.babygoodies.com
Customer Service: 845-658-9808
Gifts and baby slankets.

Baby Heirlooms
Website: http://www.babyheirlooms.com
Customer Service: 800-340-8838
Toys, clothing, and gifts.

Baby Land / Baby Land Kids Room
Website: http://www.babyland-kidsroom.com
Customer Service: 888-316-8952
Bedding, baby gear, feeding, safety, and gifts.

Baby Navigator
Website: http://www.babynavigator.com
Customer Service: online form
Safety, bedding, feeding, toys, baby care, gear, clothing, books.

Baby Net Center
Website: http://www.babynetcenter.com
Customer Service: online form
Clothing, bedding, feeding, baby gear, baby care, books, gifts.

Baby oh Baby
Website: http://www.baby-oh-baby.com
Customer Service: 800-825-4901
Feeding and gifts.

Baby Plaque
Website: http://www.babyplaque.com
Customer Service: info@babyplaque.com
Gifts.

Baby Products Online
Website: http://www.babyproductsonline.com
Customer Service: 626-914-9905
Gifts, toys, bedding, and baby gear.

Baby Secrets Online
Website: http://www.babysecretsonline.com
Customer Service: 877-818-4800
Baby care and gifts.

Baby Shower
Website: http://www.baby-shower.com
Customer Service: online form
Announcements, parenting, books/music, and gifts.

Baby Shower Gifts.com
Website: http://www.babyshowergifts.com
Customer Service: 877-638-6464
Unique gifts.

Baby Shower Mall
Website: http://www.babyshowermall.com
Customer Service: 888-831-6243
Baby gear, bedding, and gifts.

Baby Style
Website: http://www.babystyle.com
Customer Service: 877-ESTYLES
Bedding, toys, clothing, baby gear, baby care, and gifts.

Baby Suite
Website: http://www.babysuite.com
Customer Service: 877-417-BABY
Gift baskets.

Baby Supermall
Website: http://www.babysupermall.com
Customer Service: online form
Baby care, feeding, toys, bedding, clothing, safety, and gifts.

Baby T's
Website: http://www.babyts.com
Customer Service: 800-3BABYTs Fax: 530-885-0726
Clothing and gifts.

Baby Toy Town
Website: http://www.babytoytown.com
Customer Service: 626-288-6220
Toys, bedding, baby gear, and gifts.

Baby Trophy
Website: http://www.babytrophy.com
Customer Service: webmaster@babytrophy.com
Baby trophies with birth information on plaque.

Baby Universe
Website: http://www.babyuniverse.com
Customer Service: 877-615-BABY Fax: 954-523-9881
Safety, feeding, books/music, baby care, gear, toys, bedding.

Baby's Box of Treasures
Website: http://www.bbtreasures.com
Customer Service: 866-966-2229
Unique baby gifts.

Baby's Heaven
Website: http://www.babysheaven.com
Customer Service: 866-343-2836
Toys, bedding, health/safety, baby care, gear, gifts.

BabyAge.com
Website: http://www.babyage.com
Customer Service: 800-BABYAGE
Bedding, feeding, baby care, gear, gifts, safety.

Babynet Center
Website: http://www.babynetcenter.com
Customer Service: online form
Books/music, clothing, feeding, bedding, toys, baby gear.

Barney for Baby
Website: http://www.barneyforbaby.com
Customer Service: 800-418-2371
Barney clothing, books, music, toys, gifts, etc.

Bronze Cobbler
Website: http://www.bronzecobbler.com
Customer Service: 719-227-7934 Fax: 719-633-1587
Baby shoe bronzing.

Candy Bouquet & More
Website: http://www.candybouquetandmore.com
Customer Service: 866-252-6587
Gift baskets.

Charmed I'm Sure
Website: http://www.charmedimsure.net
Customer Service: 919-873-9335 Fax: 919-876-2419
Baby gifts.

Christian Expression
Website: http://www.christianexpression.com
Customer Service: 401-942-3929 Fax: 401-944-0913
Personalized products, books/music, and gifts.

Cookie Baby Inc.
Website: http://www.cookiebabyinc.com
Customer Service: 877-787-0088
Personalized baby products - toys, bedding and gifts.

Custom Baby Gifts
Website: http://www.custombabygifts.com
Customer Service: 256-890-0739
Customized gifts.

E Baby Station
Website: http://ebabystation.com
Customer Service: 706-863-4452 Fax: 706-863-4452
Bedding, gifts, pregnancy, baby care, gear, clothing, and toys.

EStyle
Website: http://www.estyle.com
Customer Service: 877-ESTYLES
Bedding, toys, clothing, pregnancy, gifts, and baby gear.

Everlasting Treasures
Website: http://www.everlastingtreasures.com
Customer Service: 866-537-3832 Fax: 928-537-3842
Hand casting kits.

Family Heirlooms
Website: http://www.familyheirlooms.com
Customer Service: 800-672-0861
Baby shoe bronzing.

First Registry
Website: http://www.firstregistry.com
Customer Service: 650-594-4387 Fax: 707-715-7696
Gift guides.

Free Gifts for Kids
Website: http://www.freegifts4kids.com
Customer Service: 916-344-3966 Fax: 916-643-0300
Present and expectant parents receive FREE gifts.

From the Womb
Website: http://www.fromthewomb.com
Customer Service: 805-528-7807
Gift baskets.

Genius Baby
Website: http://www.geniusbaby.com
Customer Service: 704-573-4500 Fax: 704-545-5716
Baby gifts, books and toys.

Gifts for Baby
Website: http://www.giftsforbaby.com
Customer Service: 201-493-8722
Clothing, toys, and gifts.

Great Beginnings
Website: http://www.childrensfurniture.com
Customer Service: 800-886-7099
Bedding/furniture, baby gear, toys, safety, books/music, and gifts.

Havoc Publishing
Website: http://www.havocpub.com
Customer Service: 858-638-8211
Unique gifts.

I Baby Doc
Website: http://www.ibabydoc.com
Customer Service: 888-758-0272
Baby care, baby gear, health/safety, and gifts.

Kid Fancies
Website: http://www.kidfancies.com
Customer Service: 877-376-2992
Distinctive furnishings and gifts for children.

Lambs and Ivy
Website: http://www.lambsivy.com
Customer Service: 800-34-LAMBS
Bedding, gifts, and safety.

Lil' Baby Cakes
Website: http://www.lilbabycakes.com
Customer Service: questions@lilbabycakes.com
Gifts.

Lillian Vernon Kids
Website: http://www.lillianvernon.com
Customer Service: 800-285-555
Toys, gifts - personalization available.

Little Bobby Creations
Website: http://www.littlebobbycreations.com
Customer Service: 219-662-6368
Personalized gift cards and baby room décor.

Little Forest
Website: http://www.littleforest.com
Customer Service: 888-329-2229
Gifts.

Little Things Mean A Lot
Website: http://www.littlethingsmeanalot.com
Customer Service: 800-333-6036
Gifts and special occasion clothing.

Lullaby Shoppe
Website: http://www.lullabyshoppe.com
Customer Service: 509-935-8809
Gift baskets and lullaby music.

Maternity Skin Care
Website: http://www.maternityskincare.com
Customer Service: 800-690-2164
Gifts and health.

Mommy Magic
Website: http://www.mommymagic.com
Customer Service: thestaff@mommymagic.com
Books, music, gifts.

My Baby Connection
Website: http://www.mybabyconnection.com
Customer Service: webmaster@mybabyconnection.com
Announcements, clothing, gifts, books, etc.

My Baby Shops
Website: http://www.mybabyshops.com
Customer Service: dawn@mybabyshops.com
Announcements, clothing, gifts, food, and much more.

Neat Stuff Gifts
Website: http://www.neatstuffgifts.com
Customer Service: 800-586-9278 Fax: 732-846-9796
Gifts, toys, and bedding.

Pampering Boutique
Website: http://www.pamperingboutique.com
Customer Service: 765-449-8514 Fax: same
Baby care, gifts, and clothing.

Parenting Concepts
Website: http://www.parentingconcepts.com
Customer Service: 800-727-3683
Baby gear, books and music, parenting, toys, and gifts.

Personalized Baby Gifts
Website: http://www.personalizedbabygifts.com
Customer Service: service@personalizedbabygifts.com
Announcements and gifts.

Picture Perfect Baby
Website: http://www.pictureperfectbaby.com
Customer Service: 877-621-BABY Fax: 919-469-3490
Announcements, baby names, and gifts.

Poshtots
Website: http://www.poshtots.com
Customer Service: 866-POSH-TOTS Fax:804-935-0844
Bedding and gifts.

Pottery Barn Kids
Website: http://www.potterybarnkids.com
Customer Service: 888-779-5176 Fax: 702-363-2541
Bedding, furniture, and gifts.

Rich Frog 📖
Website: http://www.richfrog.com
Customer Service: webinfo@richfrog.com
Toys, gifts, and baby care.

Ring Box
Website: http://www.ringbox.com
Customer Service: 888-646-6466
Gifts.

Ritzy Rascals
Website: http://ritzyrascals.com
Customer Service: 866-URASCAL
Clothing and gifts.

Royal Baby
Website: http://www.royalbaby.com
Customer Service: 866-855-1945 Fax: 309-416-4472
Parenting, pregnancy, clothing, toys, gifts, etc.

Royal Nursery, The
Website: http://www.newborngifts.com
Customer Service: 858-450-1317
Gifts, music, baby care, bedding, clothing, books.

Russ Berrie & Company
Website: http://www.russberrie.com
Customer Service: 800-358-8278
Plush toys, gifts, and bedding accessories.

Shopping Galore
Website: http://www.shoppinggalore.com/Babiesgalore.html
Customer Service: 866-517-9608 Fax: 662-513-6667
Toys, gifts, and much more.

Stork Avenue
Website: http://www.storkavenue.com
Customer Service: 800-861-5437
Baby announcements and gifts.

Stork Delivers, The
Website: http://www.thestorkdelivers.com
Customer Service: 800-94-BABYS
Gift baskets, bedding, and announcements.

Sure Baby
Website: http://www.surebaby.com
Customer Service: customercare@surebaby.com
Pregnancy, gifts, and baby care.

Sweet Pea Company
Website: http://www.sweetpeacompany.com
Customer Service: online form
Gifts, bedding, music, and parenting.

Target Lullaby Club
Website: http://www.target.com
Customer Service: 800-888-9333
Everything baby.

Teddy Luv
Website: http://www.teddyluv.com
Customer Service: 877-HUG-7577
Personalized teddy bear gifts.

Tooth Fairy Central
Website: http://www.toothfairycentral.com
Customer Service: 800-441-7340
Toothfairy gifts, pillows, boxes and bears.

Toys R Us
Website: http://www.toysrus.com
Customer Service: 800-TOYS-R-Us
Toys, feeding, baby care, gear,bedding/furniture, books/music.

Treasured Baby Steps
Website: http://www.treasuredbabysteps.com
Customer Service: 877-821-0060
Personalized porcelain baby shoes.

Wee Snuggles
Website: http://www.weesnuggles.com
Customer Service: 866-665-8631
Announcements and gifts.

Wish World
Website: http://www.wishworld.com
Customer Service: online form
Gift registry.

Health and Safety

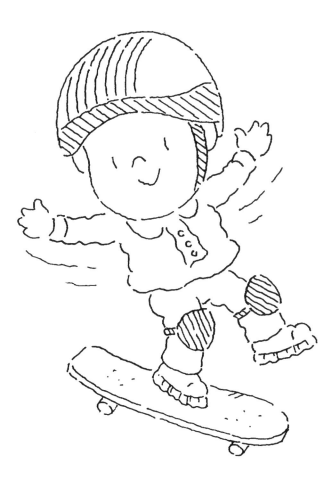

Able Baby
Website: http://www.ablebaby.com
Customer Service: ablebabyco@aol.com
Safety, baby care, bedding, books/music/videos, toys.

Answer for Colic
Website: http://www.answer-for-colic.com
Customer Service: 800-270-7539
Tips for handling a colicy baby.

Babies Planet
Website: http://www.thebabiesplanet.com
Customer Service: susan@thebabuesplanet.com
Parenting, baby care, health, pregnancy, baby foods, and names.

Babies-R-Us
Website: http://www.babiesrus.com
Customer Service: 800-BABYRUS
Everything baby.

Baby Abby
Website: http://www.babyabby.com
Customer Service: 800-972-7357 Fax: 303-777-6117
Baby care, gear, clothing, pregnancy, safety, gifts.

Baby Ant
Website: http://www.babyant.com
Customer Service: online form
Toys, clothing, health, bedding, and gifts.

Baby Bag Online
Website: http://www.babybag.com
Customer Service: 949-388-5257
Baby gear, announcements, pregnancy, parenting, safety, feeding.

Baby Bottle Safety Information Center
Website: http://www.babybottle.org
Customer Service: webmaster@babybottle.org
Feeding safety tips.

Baby Buddy
Website: http://www.babybuddy.com
Customer Service: 877-382-1010
Baby care and safety.

Baby Chatter
Website: http://www.babychatter.com
Customer Service: info@babychatter.com
Baby names, safety, books, and announcements.

Baby Land
Website: http://www.babyland.com
Customer Service: stork@babyland.com
Announcements, books, and parenting.

Baby Land / Baby Land Kids Room
Website: http://www.babyland-kidsroom.com
Customer Service: 888-316-8952
Bedding, baby gear, feeding, safety, and gifts.

Baby Lounge
Website: http://www.babylounge.com
Customer Service: 973-921-0852
Parenting, pregnancy, announcements, health/safety.

Baby Med
Website: http://www.babymed.com
Customer Service: support@babymed.com
Health and pregnancy.

Baby Mountain
Website: http://www.babymountain.com
Customer Service: mail@babymountain.com
Announcements, clothing, feeding, names, toys, safety, bedding.

Baby Needs
Website: http://www.babyneeds.com
Customer Service: 800-672-5313
Parenting, feeding, and health/safety.

Baby News Online
Website: http://www.babynewsonline.com
Customer Service: 866-437-BABY
Bedding, baby gear, baby care, feeding, health/safety.

Baby Place
Website: http://www.baby-place.com
Customer Service: online form
Health/safety, parenting, pregnancy, and toys.

Baby Pro
Website: http://www.babypro.com
Customer Service: 800-859-0657
Child proofing products.

Baby Proofing
Website: http://www.babyproofing.com
Customer Service: 888-494-7111
Baby-proofing your home.

Baby Proofing Plus
Website: http://www.babyproofingplus.com
Customer Service: 800-683-7233 Fax: 905-761-0857
Baby-proofing.

Baby Resource
Website: http://www.babyresource.com
Customer Service: online form
Toys, health/safety, and books/music.

Baby Safe and Sound
Website: http://www.babysafeandsound.com
Customer Service: 877-939-2229 Fax: 310-450-0143
Help make your home safe.

Baby Supermall
Website: http://www.babysupermall.com
Customer Service: online form
Baby care, feeding, toys, bedding, clothing, safety, and gifts.

Baby Tips
Website: http://www.babytips.co.uk
Customer Service: UK
Feeding, pregnancy, health/safety, and parenting.

Baby Universe
Website: http://www.babyuniverse.com
Customer Service: 877-615-BABY Fax: 954-523-9881
Safety, feeding, books/music, baby care, gear, toys, bedding.

Baby's Doc
Website: http://www.babysdoc.com
Customer Service: 727-459-4277
Health and safety.

Baby's Heaven
Website: http://www.babysheaven.com
Customer Service: 866-343-2836
Toys, bedding, health/safety, baby care, gear, gifts.

BabyAge.com
Website: http://www.babyage.com
Customer Service: 800-BABYAGE
Bedding, feeding, baby care, gear, gifts, safety.

Basic Comfort
Website: http://www.basiccomfort.com
Customer Service: 800-456-8687
Bedding, clothing, baby care, and health/safety.

Carolina Baby
Website: http://www.carolinababy.com
Customer Service: dawn@babyuniversity.com
Baby care, pregnancy, baby names, parenting, health/safety.

Chicken Pox Info
Website: http://www.chickenfoxinfo.com
Customer Service: online form
Information on Chicken Pox.

Child Safe Pool Fence
Website: http://www.childsafepoolfence.com
Customer Service: 813-249-6309
Child safe fences for pools.

Child Safety Products
Website: http://www.materialsforpackaging.com/child
Customer Service: 800-841-5903
Safety.

Cryobank Cord Blood Services
Website: http://www.cryobank.com/baby
Customer Service:800-233373 Fax: 310-443-5258
Health.

Cryo-cell International Inc.
Website: http://www.cryo-cell.com
Customer Service: 800-STOR-CELL
Health.

Curad
Website: http://www.curadusa.com
Customer Service: online form
First aid supplies.

Danny Foundation
Website: http://www.dannyfoundation.org
Customer Service: 800-83DANNY
Baby crib and child product safety.

E Baby Superstore
Website: http://www.ebabysuperstore.com
Customer Service: 877-253-7717 Fax: 425-357-1856
Toys, safety, baby care, baby gear, books/music.

Earplanes
Website: http://www.earplanes.com
Customer Service: 800-327-6151
Earplugs for children that fly.

Express Baby
Website: http://www.expressbaby.com
Customer Service: 800-600-0410
Baby care, gear, feeding, bedding, gifts, safety, and clothing.

Fit Pregnancy
Website: http://ww2.fitpregnancy-1.com
Customer Service: online form
Health and pregnancy.

For Babies
Website: http://www.4babies.com
Customer Service: 510-768-1444
Books, parenting, clothing, safety and baby names.

Great Beginnings
Website: http://www.childrensfurniture.com
Customer Service: 800-886-7099
Bedding/furniture, baby gear, toys, safety, books/music, and gifts.

Healthy Kids
Website: http://www.healthykids.com
Customer Service: online form
Health.

I Baby Doc
Website: http://www.ibabydoc.com
Customer Service: 888-758-0272
Baby care, baby gear, health/safety, and gifts.

Johnson & Johnson Pediatric Institute
Website: http://www.jjpi.com
Customer Service: 877-JNJ-LINK
Health site full of information.

Keep Kids Healthy
Website: http://www.keepkidshealthy.com/baby.html
Customer Service: online forms
Health.

Kidalog
Website: http://www.kidalog.com
Customer Service: 780-672-1763 Fax: 780-672-6942
Clothing, safety, breast pumps, and much more.

KidCo Inc.
Website: http://www.kidcoinc.com
Customer Service: 800-553-5529
Baby gear and safety.

Kiddopotamus
Website: http://www.kiddopotamus.com
Customer Service: 800-772-8339
Baby gear and safety.

Kids Health
Website: http://www.kidshealth.org
Customer Service: online form
Health and education for parents.

Lambs and Ivy
Website: http://www.lambsivy.com
Customer Service: 800-34-LAMBS
Bedding, gifts, and safety.

Leachco
Website: http://www.leachco.com
Customer Service: 800-525-1050
Bedding, baby care, health/safety, baby gear, and pregnancy.

Little Remedies
Website: http://www.littleremedies.com
Customer Service: 800-7-LITTLE
Health.

Maternity Skin Care
Website: http://www.maternityskincare.com
Customer Service: 800-690-2164
Gifts and health.

Mayo Health
Website: http://www.mayohealth.org
Customer Service: online form
Health.

Mead Johnson Nutritionals
Website: http://www.meadjohnson.com
Customer Service: 812-439-5000
Health and baby food.

Medem
Website: http://www.medem.com
Customer Service: 877-926-3336
Health.

My Medcab
Website: http://www.mymedcab.com
Customer Service: 877-TYLENOL
Medicine cabinet essentials.

Mylicon
Website: http://www.mylicon.com
Customer Service: 800-222-9435
Medicine/Health.

Marrott Baby Products
Website: http://www.babyproductsstore.com
Customer Service: service@babyproductstore.com
Baby gear and safety.

National Conference on Shaken Baby Syndrome
Website: http://www.dontshake.com
Customer Service: 888-273-0071 Fax: 801-627-3321
Health.

Natural Baby
Website: http://www.naturalbaby.com
Customer Service: 800-388-BABY
Health.

Natural Mom
Website: http://www.naturalmom.com
Customer Service: 608-242-0200
Health, pregnancy, books, and baby care.

Noel Joanna, Inc. (NoJo)
Website: http://www.nojo.com
Customer Service: 800-85408760
Safety, furniture, and bedding.

Nurse Donna's Baby Land
Website: http://www.123babyland.com
Customer Service: 800-894-0289
Books/music/videos, safety, and baby care.

Nursery Bright
Website: http://www.nurserybright.com
Customer Service: 877-BABY-959
Baby care, furniture, bedding, safety, clothing and gear.

Nursery Rhymes
Website: http://www.nurseryrhymes.com
Customer Service: 519-743-1321 Fax: 519-743-1681
Baby gear, furniture/bedding, toys, and safety.

One Step Ahead
Website: http://www.onestepahead.com
Customer Service: 800-274-8440
Clothing, baby care, gear, safety, pregnancy, and more.

Orajel
Website: http://www.orajel.com
Customer Service: 800-952-5080
Health.

Parent Stages
Website: http://www.parentstages.com
Customer Service: online form
Parenting and health.

Perfectly Safe
Website: http://www.perfectlysafe.com
Customer Service: 800-837-5437
Safety and books.

Play Fence
Website: http://www.playfence.com
Customer Service: 800-242-8190 Fax: 941-639-7488
Safety gates.

Pregnant Inc.
Website: http://www.pregnantinc.com
Customer Service: 626-288-6220
Bedding, furniture, and baby gear.

Pregnancy
Website: http://www.women.com/pregnancy
Customer Service: online form
Parenting, pregnancy, babycare, and safety.

Prince Lionheart
Website: http://www.princelionheart.com
Customer Service: 800-544-1132 Fax: 805-982-9442
Bedding, baby care, and safety.

Red Calliope
Website: http://www.redcalliope.com
Customer Service: 800-421-0526
Safety, bedding, maternity, and baby care.

Revital Online
Website: http://www.revitalonline.com
Customer Service: 800-789-1515
Health.

Safe Kids
Website: http://safekids.com
Customer Service: info@safekids.com
Safety.

Safe Kids
Website: http://www.safekids.org
Customer Service: 202-662-0600 Fax: 202-393-2072
Safety.

Safety 1st
Website: http://www.safety1st.com
Customer Service: 800-723-3065
Safety, baby gear, and baby food.

Security and More
Website: http://www.securityandmore.com
Customer Service: 800-444-6278
Safety, high-tech baby monitors.

Storkcraft
Website: http://www.storkcraft.com
Customer Service: 604-275-4242 Fax: 604-274-9727
Furniture and safety.

Target Lullaby Club
Website: http://www.target.com
Customer Service: 800-888-9333
Everything baby.

Toys R Us
Website: http://www.toysrus.com
Customer Service: 800-TOYS-R-Us
Toys, feeding, baby care, gear,bedding/furniture, books/music.

Tylenol
Website: http://www.tylenol.com
Customer Service: 800-962-5357
Health.

UK Mother
Website: http://www.ukmother.com
Customer Service: UK
Pregnancy, health, baby gear.

Very Best Baby
Website: http://www.verybestbaby.com
Customer Service: 800-456-6035
Health, food, parenting, and more.

Viacord
Website: http://www.viacord.com
Customer Service: 866-565-2221
Cord blood preservation - Health.

Yellow Dyno
Website: http://www.yellowdyno.com
Customer Service: 888-954-KIDS
Tips on how to safely raising children.

Your Amazing Baby
Website: http://www.amazingbaby.com
Customer Service: kellyr@amazingbaby.com
Parenting, feeding, and health/safety.

Parenting

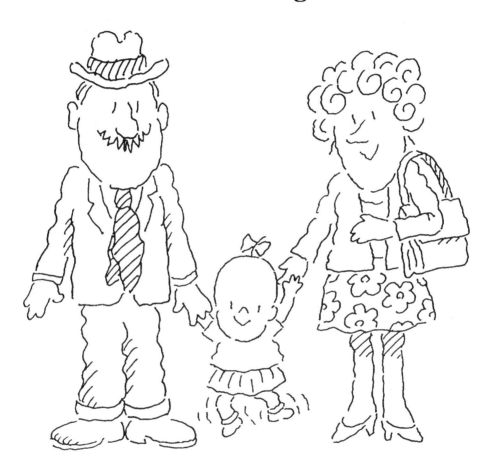

A Baby Made
Website: http://www.ababymade.com
Customer Service: online form
Fertility and Adoption grants.

ABC Baby
Website: http://abcbaby.org
Customer Service: mail@abcbaby.org
Baby products guide.

Babies Planet
Website: http://www.thebabiesplanet.com
Customer Service: susan@thebabiesplanet.com
Parenting, baby care, health, pregnancy, baby foods, names.

Babies-R-Us
Website: http://www.babiesrus.com
Customer Service: 800-BABYRUS
Everything baby- Baby Superstore.

Baby Bag Online
Website: http://www.babybag.com
Customer Service: 949-388-5257
Baby gear, announcements, pregnancy, parenting, safety, feeding.

Baby Center
Website: http://www.babycenter.com
Customer Service: online form
Parenting, pregnancy, announcements, baby gear, and safety.

Baby Corner, The
Website: http://www.thebabycorner.com
Customer Service: 812-867-3759
Baby care, pregnancy, parenting, gear, clothing, toys, bedding.

Baby Daily
Website: http://www.babydaily.com
Customer Service: 847-556-2300 Fax: 847-424-9821
Pregnancy, parenting, breastfeeding, and baby care.

Baby Knows Best
Website: http://www.babyknowsbest.com
Customer Service: info@babyknowsbest.com
Parenting.

Baby Lounge
Website: http://www.babylounge.com
Customer Service: 973-921-0852
Parenting, pregnancy, announcements, health/safety.

Baby n' Mom
Website: http://www.baby-n-mom.com
Customer Service: webmaster@best-toys-prices.com
Clothing, bedding, parenting, names, and baby gear.

Baby Needs
Website: http://www.babyneeds.com
Customer Service: 800-672-5313
Parenting, feeding, and health/safety.

Baby Online
Website: http://www.babyonline.com
Customer Service: London
Parenting, baby care, toys, and feeding.

Baby Parenting
Website: http://babyparenting.about.com
Customer Service: 212-204-4000
Parenting.

Baby Place
Website: http://www.baby-place.com
Customer Service: online form
Health/safety, parenting, pregnancy, and toys.

Baby Scapes
Website: http://www.babyscapes.com
Customer Service: 888-441-KIDS
Parenting and books/music.

Baby Shower
Website: http://www.baby-shower.com
Customer Service: online form
Announcements, parenting, books/music, and gifts.

Baby Signs
Website: http://www.babysigns.com
Customer Service: 800-995-0226
Parenting and books/music.

Baby Talk
Website: http://www.babytalk.com
Customer Service: online form
Parenting magazine.

Baby Tips
Website: http://www.babytips.co.uk
Customer Service: UK
Feeding, pregnancy, health/safety, and parenting.

Baby Travel Solutions
Website: http://www.babytravelsolutions.com
Customer Service: 888-989-0302 Fax: 303-428-7479
Order what you need and it will be waiting for you on your trip.

Baby Zone
Website: http://www.babyzone.com
Customer Service: webmaster@babyzone.com
Baby names, parenting, announcements, and pregnancy.

Baby's Play
Website: http://www.babysplay.com
Customer Service: 402-895-7984
Parenting and pregnancy.

Carnation
Website: http://www.carnationbaby.com
Customer Service: 800-CARNATION
Parenting, pregnancy, baby food and formula.

Carolina Baby
Website: http://www.carolinababy.com
Customer Service: dawn@babyuniversity.com
Baby care, pregnancy, names, parenting, health/safety.

Cherished Moments
Website: http://www.cherishedmoments.com
Customer Service: 713-957-2764 Fax: 713-957-2764
Toys, bedding, parenting, names, and baby gear.

Child Care Aware Organization
Website: http://www.childcareaware.org
Customer Service: 800-424-2246
Tips on finding child care.

Child Development Web
Website: http://www.childdevelopmentweb.com
Customer Service: 718-351-0518
Pregnancy and parenting.

Club Mom
Website: http://www.clubmom.com
Customer Service: 646-435-6500 Fax: 646-435-6600
Parenting.

College Savings
Website: http://www.collegesavings.org
Customer Service: 877-277-6496
Information about 529 State College Savings plans.

Education
Website: http://www.education.com
Customer Service: 800-545-7677
Parenting and books.

Educating Baby
Website: http://www.educatingbaby.com
Customer Service: 800-533-5392
Parenting and books.

Enfamil
Website: http://www.enfamil.com
Customer Service: 800 BABY-123
Baby formula and parenting guides.

Family Labels
Website: http://www.familylabels.com
Customer Service: 800-284-6192
Unique family address labels.

Family Life Magazine
Website: http://www.familylifmag.com
Customer Service: 800-682-7667
Parenting and magazines.

Family Web
Website: http://www.familyweb.com
Customer Service: 650-462-9019
Pregnancy and parenting.

For Babies
Website: http://www.4babies.com
Customer Service: 510-768-1444
Books, parenting, clothing, safety and baby names.

Gentle Mom
Website: http://www.gentlemom.com
Customer Service: 877-833-BABY
Baby gear, baby care, books/music, and parenting.

Goodnites
Website: http://www.goodnites.com
Customer Service: 920-721-2553 Fax: 920-721-2035
Disposable absorbant underpants and potty training tips.

Growing Child
Website: http://www.growingchild.com
Customer Service: 800-927-7289
Child development newsletter.

Having a Baby Today
Website: http://www.havingababytoday.com
Customer Service: 800-743-0974 Fax: 541-344-1422
Pregnancy, breastfeeding, and parenting.

Having Another Baby
Website: http://www.havinganotherbaby.com
Customer Service: 516-944-5856 Fax: 516-621-8310
Parenting and pregnancy.

Hi Baby
Website: http://www.hibaby.com
Customer Service: 888-HIBABY9
Preemie website, clothing, and baby contests.

Huggies Supreme
Website: http://www.parentstages.com
Customer Service: 800-544-1847
Baby care and parenting tips.

Innovative Parents
Website: http://www.innovative-parents.com
Customer Service: 888-252-5437
Parenting.

Jewelry by Kelly Colleen
Website: http://www.jewelrybykellycolleen.com
Customer Service: 800-435-1426
Mommy Bracelets.

Kids in Mind
Website: http://www.kids-in-mind.com
Customer Service: 513-761-1188
Movie reviews with kids in mind.

Labor of Love, The
Website: http://www.thelaboroflove.com
Customer Service: webmaster@thelaboroflove.com
Pregnancy and parenting

Learn Free Parenting
Website: http://www.learnfree-parenting.com
Customer Service: online form
Pregnancy and parenting.

Making Lemonade
Website: http://www.makinglemonade.com
Customer Service: jody@makinglemonade.com
Parenting.

Maternity Mall
Website: http://www.maternitymall.com
Customer Service: online form
Maternity, pregnancy, and parenting.

Memphis Parent
Website: http://www.memphisparent.com
Customer Service: mphsparent@contemporary-media.com
Parenting.

Mom Shop
Website: http://www.momshop.com
Customer Service: 800-854-1213
Clothing, maternity, pregnancy, parenting.

Mom's Love, A
Website: http://www.amomslove.com
Customer Service: online form
Parenting, magazine.

My Little Steps
Website: http://www.mylittlesteps.com
Customer Service: customercare@mylittlesteps.com
Parenting and education.

Natural Baby Info
Website: http://www.naturalbabyinfo.com
Customer Service: webmaster@naturalbabyinfo.com
Parenting.

Nursing Baby
Website: http://www.nursingbaby.com
Customer Service: 979-569-8528
Parenting and nursing.

Nurtured Baby
Website: http://www.nurturedbaby.com
Customer Service: 888-564-BABY
Nursing and parenting.

Pampers
Website: http://www.pampers.com
Customer Service: 800-PAMPERS
Diapers and parenting.

Parent and Baby
Website: http://www.townonline.com/parentandbaby
Customer Service: 877-CNC-BABY Fax: 781-453-6610
Parenting.

Parent Hub
Website: http://www.parenthub.com
Customer Service: info@parenthub.com
Parenting, clothing, funiture, toys, and books.

Parent Stages
Website: http://www.parentstages.com
Customer Service: online form
Parenting and health.

Parent to be Calendar
Website: http://www.2bparent.com/calendar
Customer Service: 954-782-8668 Fax: 954-782-9656
Parenting and pregnancy videos.

Parenthood Web
Website: http://www.parenthoodweb.com
Customer Service: online fom
Parenting.

Parenting
Website: http://www.parenting.com
Customer Service: online fom
Parenting magazine.

Parenting Concepts
Website: http://www.parentingconcepts.com
Customer Service: 800-727-3683
Baby gear, books/music, parenting, toys, and gifts.

Parenting Humor
Website: http://www.parentinghumor.com
Customer Service: editor@parentinghumor.com
Paenting humor.

Parenting Place
Website: http://www.parentingplace.com
Customer Service: webmaster@parentingplace.com
Parenting.

Parents Without Partners
Website: http://www.parentswithoutpartners.org
Customer Service: 800-637-7974
Parenting.

PBS Kids
Website: http://www.pbskids.org
Customer Service: 703-739-5000
Parenting and games.

Pregnancy
Website: http://www.women.com/pregnancy
Customer Service: online form
Parenting, pregnancy, babycare, and safety.

Professor Mom
Website: http://www.professormom.com
Customer Service: 503-630-3542
Educational site.

PTA
Website: http://www.pta.org
Customer Service: 800-307-4PTA Fax: 312-670-6783
Parenting magazine.

Pull Ups
Website: http://www.pullups.com
Customer Service: online form
Baby care and parenting.

Royal Baby
Website: http://www.royalbaby.com
Customer Service: 866-855-1945 Fax: 309-416-4472
Parenting, pregnancy, clothing, toys, gifts, etc.

Scholastic
Website: http://www.scholastic.com
Customer Service: online form
Parenting and books.

Sesame Street
Website: http://www.sesamestreet.com
Customer Service: online form
Stories, games, parenting, music, pregnancy, etc.

Sesame Street Workshop
Website: http://www.sesameworkshop.org
Customer Service: online form
Stories, games, parenting, music, pregnancy, etc

Sign to Me
Website: http://www.sign2me.com
Customer Service: 206-361-0307 Fax: 206-362-2025
Learn to communicate with your baby through sign language.

Similac
Website: http://www.similac.com
Customer Service: 800-227-5767
Parenting and baby formula.

Single Mothers By Choice
Website: http://www.singlemothersbychoice.com
Customer Service: 212-988-0993
Parenting.

Sleep Baby
Website: http://www.sleepbaby.com
Customer Service: 888-795-0555
Parenting, videos.

Snibbie
Website: http://www.snibbie.com
Customer Service: 202-508-3673 Fax: 202-331-3759
Adult bibs - protect your clothing from baby stains.

Sweet Pea Company
Website: http://www.sweetpeacompany.com
Customer Service: online form
Gifts, bedding, music, and parenting.

Target Lullaby Club
Website: http://www.target.com
Customer Service: 800-888-9333
Everything baby.

TL Care
Website: http://www.tlcare.com
Customer Service: online form
Baby care, parenting, and nursing products.

Toys R Us
Website: http://www.toysrus.com
Customer Service: 800-TOYS-R-Us
Toys, feeding, baby care, gear,bedding/furniture, books/music.

Twins Magazine
Website: http://www.twinsmagazine.com
Customer Service: 888-558-9467
Twin and pregnancy information.

U.S. Consumer Products Safety Commission
Website: http://www.cpsc.gov
Customer Service: 800-638-2772
Parenting and baby gear.

UPROMISE
Website: http://www.upromise.com
Customer Service:
Start saving for college for your baby.

Very Best Baby
Website: http://www.verybestbaby.com
Customer Service: 800-456-6035
Health, food, parenting, and more.

Working Mother Magazine
Website: http://www.workingmother.com
Customer Service: Online form
Parenting advice for working mothers.

You and Your Child
Website: http://www.tesco.com/youandyourchild
Customer Service: UK
Pregnancy, parenting, feeding, and baby care.

Your Amazing Baby
Website: http://www.amazingbaby.com
Customer Service: kellyr@amazingbaby.com
Parenting, feeding, and health/safety.

Your Baby Today
Website: http://www.yourbabytoday.com
Customer Service: online form
Pregnancy and parenting.

Pregnancy, Breastfeeding, and Maternity.

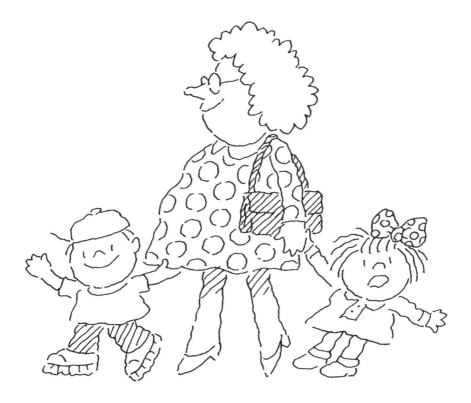

A Baby Made
Website: http://www.ababymade.com
Customer Service: online form
Fertility and Adoption grants.

Alternative Baby
Website: http://www.alternativebaby.com
Customer Service: 800-469-1126
Baby care, gear, clothing, pregnancy, toys, and gifts baskets.

American Baby Company
Website: http://www.americanbaby.com
Customer Service: 909-597-9070
Clothing, toys, pregnancy, parenting, and gifts.

Annacris
Website: http://www.annacris.com
Customer Service: 800-281-ANNA
Maternity clothing.

Attachments 📖
Website: http://www.attachmentscatalog.com
Customer Service: 800-873-5023
Toys, breastfeeding, gifts, books, and baby gear.

Avent America, Inc.
Website: http://www.aventamerica.com
Customer Service: 800-542-8368
Bottles, breast pumps, skin care, and pacifiers.

Babies Online
Website: http://www.babiesonline.com
Customer Service: online form
Pregnancy.

Babies Planet
Website: http://www.thebabiesplanet.com
Customer Service: susan@thebabuesplanet.com
Parenting, baby care, health, pregnancy, baby foods, and names.

Babies-R-Us
Website: http://www.babiesrus.com
Customer Service: 800-BABYRUS
Everything baby.

Babies Today
Website: http://babiestoday.com
Customer Service: 847-556-2300 Fax: 847-424-9821
Pregnancy and breastfeeding.

Baby Bag Online
Website: http://www.babybag.com
Customer Service: 949-388-5257
Baby gear, announcements, pregnancy, parenting, safety, feeding.

Baby Bargains
Website: http://www.babybargains.com
Customer Service: 540-899-6090
Toys, pregnancy, and clothing.

Baby Becoming 📖
Website: http://www.babybecoming.com
Customer Service: 888-666-6910
Maternity and nursing clothing.

Baby Best Buy
Website: http://www.babybestbuy.com
Customer Service: 877-BABY-BUY
Bedding, baby care, and feeding/breastfeeding.

Baby Boom
Website: http://www.babyboom1.com
Customer Service: 800-929-4666
Gifts, pregnancy, clothing, and toys.

Baby Care
Website: http://babycare-sa.com
Customer Service: 866-343-2836
Baby gear, bedding, gifts, nursing, toys, and more.

Baby Center
Website: http://www.babycenter.com
Customer Service: online form
Parenting, pregnancy, announcements, baby gear, and safety.

Baby Corner, The
Website: http://www.thebabycorner.com
Customer Service: 812-867-3759
Baby care, pregnancy, parenting, gear, clothing, toys, bedding.

Baby Daily
Website: http://www.babydaily.com
Customer Service: 847-556-2300 Fax: 847-424-9821
Pregnancy, parenting, breastfeeding, and baby care.

Baby Estore
Website: http://www.babyestore.com
Customer Service: 866-580-BABY
Breastfeeding supplies, bedding, and gifts.

Baby Gap
Website: http://www.babygap.com
Customer Service: 800-427-7895
Clothing for baby, children, and expectant mothers.

Baby Gifts 4 Less
Website: http://www.babygifts-4less.com
Customer Service: 877-378-4411
Baby gear, safety, bedding, toys, feeding, pregnancy, and gifts.

Baby Lounge
Website: http://www.babylounge.com
Customer Service: 973-921-0852
Parenting, pregnancy, announcements, health/safety.

Baby Med
Website: http://www.babymed.com
Customer Service: support@babymed.com
Health and pregnancy.

Baby Place
Website: http://www.baby-place.com
Customer Service: online form
Health/safety, parenting, pregnancy, and toys.

Baby Plus
Website: http://www.babyplus.com
Customer Service: 317-815-1111
Pregnancy.

Baby Tips
Website: http://www.babytips.co.uk
Customer Service: UK
Feeding, pregnancy, health/safety, and parenting.

Baby Zone
Website: http://www.babyzone.com
Customer Service: webmaster@babyzone.com
Names, parenting, announcements, and pregnancy.

Baby's Play
Website: http://www.babysplay.com
Customer Service: 402-895-7984
Parenting and pregnancy.

Bailey Medical Engineering
Website: http://www.baileymed.com
Customer Service: 800-413-3216
Breast pumps and supplies.

Bareware
Website: http://bareware.net
Customer Service: 877-9 DIAPER
Clothing, toys, baby care, gear, and pregnancy.

Basically Baby
Website: http://weeshop.com
Customer Service: 888-254-8780
Bedding, baby care, clothing, and pregnancy.

Belly Basics
Website: http://www.bellybasics.com
Customer Service: 800-378-9537
Pregnancy.

Belly Butter
Website: http://www.bellybutter.com
Customer Service: 800-96-BELLY
Belly Butter for reducing your stretch marks.

Birth and Baby
Website: http://www.birthandbaby.com
Customer Service: 888-398-7987
Books/music, pregnancy, and clothing.

Bon Appetit Baby
Website: http://www.bonappetitbaby.com
Customer Service: 831-728-1553 Fax: 415-723-7618
Breastfeeding.

Boppy
Website: http://www.boppy.com
Customer Service: 303-526-2626
Nursing pillows.

Bosom Buddies
Website: http://www.bosombuddies.com
Customer Service: 888-860-0041
Breastfeeding supplies.

Breast Is Best
Website: http://www.breastisbest.com
Customer Service: 425-774-9355
Breastfeeding.

Canada Baby Works
Website: http://www.canadababyworks.com
Customer Service: 877-531-BABY
Clothing, baby care, gear, toys, and pregnancy.

Carnation
Website: http://www.carnationbaby.com
Customer Service: 800-CARNATION
Parenting, pregnancy, baby food, and formula.

Carolina Baby
Website: http://www.carolinababy.com
Customer Service: dawn@babyuniversity.com
Baby care, pregnancy, names, parenting, health/safety.

Child Birth
Website: http://www.childbirth.org
Customer Service: 502-897-7664
Pregnancy and feeding.

Child Birth Class
Website: http://www.childbirthclass.com
Customer Service: 909-985-6151
Child birth classes and videos.

Child Development Web
Website: http://www.childdevelopmentweb.com
Customer Service: 718-351-0518
Pregnancy and parenting.

Comfort Living
Website: http://www.baby-store.net
Customer Service: 877-378-4411
Feeding, health/safety, baby gear, bedding, toys, pregnancy.

Dax & Coe
Website: http://www.daxandcoe.com
Customer Service: 415-356-2277
Maternity clothing.

E Baby Station
Website: http://ebabystation.com
Customer Service: 706-863-4452 Fax: 706-863-4452
Bedding, gifts, pregnancy, baby care, gear, clothing, and toys.

E Pregnancy
Website: http://www.epregnancy.com
Customer Service: 925-447-6667 Fax: 925-937-7203
Pregnancy, books, and baby names.

EStyle
Website: http://www.estyle.com
Customer Service: 877-ESTYLES
Bedding, toys, clothing, pregnancy, gifts, and baby gear.

Eco Baby
Website: http://www.ecobaby.com
Customer Service: 800-596-7450
Pregnancy, bedding, baby care, books/music, and clothing.

Elizabeth Lee Designs
Website: http://www.elizabethlee.com
Customer Service: 435-454-3350
Nursingwear.

Expressiva
Website: http://www.expressiva.com
Customer Service: 877-933-9773
Nursingwear.

Family Web
Website: http://www.familyweb.com
Customer Service: 650-462-9019
Pregnancy and parenting.

Fit Maternity 📖
Website: http://www.fitmaternity.com
Customer Service: 888-961-9100
Maternity and nursing clothing.

Fit Pregnancy
Website: http://ww2.fitpregnancy-1.com
Customer Service: online form
Health and pregnancy.

Having a Baby Today
Website: http://www.havingababytoday.com
Customer Service: 800-743-0974 Fax: 541-344-1422
Pregnancy, breastfeeding, and parenting.

Having Another Baby
Website: http://www.havinganotherbaby.com
Customer Service: 516-944-5856 Fax: 516-621-8310
Parenting and pregnancy.

I Dream of Baby
Website: http://www.idreamofbaby.com
Customer Service: service@idreamofbaby.com
Pregnancy.

I Maternity
Website: http://www.imaternity.com
Customer Service: 800-344-0011
Pregnancy and baby names.

Jake and Me
Website: http://www.jakeandme.com
Customer Service: 970-352-8802
Maternity, nursing, infant, and toddler clothing.

KBA Breast Pump Shop
Website: http://www.kba-breastpump-shop.com
Customer Service: 888-748-4225
Breast feeding information and supplies.

Kidalog
Website: http://www.kidalog.com
Customer Service: 780-672-1763 Fax: 780-672-6942
Clothing, safety, breast pumps, and much more.

Kisses From Heaven
Website: http://www.kissesfromheaven.com
Customer Service: 888-833-8697 Fax: 816-350-0253
Nursing pillows, labor comfort kits, etc.

La Leche League
Website: http://www.lalecheleague.com
Customer Service: 800-LALECHE
Breastfeeding info and products.

Labor of Love, The
Website: http://www.thelaboroflove.com
Customer Service: webmaster@thelaboroflove.com
Pregnancy and parenting

Leachco
Website: http://www.leachco.com
Customer Service: 800-525-1050
Bedding, baby care, health/safety, baby gear, and pregnancy.

Leading Lady
Website: http://www.leadinglady.com
Customer Service: 800-321-4804
Pregnancy/maternity.

Learn Free Parenting
Website: http://www.learnfree-parenting.com
Customer Service: online form
Pregnancy and parenting.

Maternity Mall
Website: http://www.maternitymall.com
Customer Service: online form
Maternity, pregnancy, and parenting.

Maternity Skin Care
Website: http://www.maternityskincare.com
Customer Service: 800-690-2164
Gifts, pregnancy, and health.

Medela
Website: http://www.medela.com
Customer Service:800-435-8316
Pregnancy and breastfeeding supplies.

Meijer Baby Club
Website: http://www.meijer.com/babyclub
Customer Service: 800-543-3704
Feeding, baby gear, bedding, baby care, pregnancy, and toys.

Mom Shop
Website: http://www.momshop.com
Customer Service: 800-854-1213
Clothing, maternity, pregnancy, parenting.

Mother Wear
Website: http://www.motherwear.com
Customer Service: 800-950-2500
Maternity and nursing wear.

Motherhood Maternity 📖
Website: http://www.motherhood.com
Customer Service: 800-4-MOM-2-BE
Maternity, nursing wear, and baby names.

Natural Mom
Website: http://www.naturalmom.com
Customer Service: 608-242-0200
Health, pregnancy, books, and baby care.

Nursing
Website: http://www.russettweb.com/nursing.html
Customer Service: 877-865-9786
Baby gear and nursing information.

Nursing Baby
Website: http://www.nursingbaby.com
Customer Service: 979-569-8528
Parenting and nursing.

Nurtured Baby
Website: http://www.nurturedbaby.com
Customer Service: 888-564-BABY
Nursing and parenting.

Old Navy
Website: http://www.oldnavy.com
Customer Service: 800-OLD-NAVY
Clothing and maternity.

One Hot Mama 📖
Website: http://www.onehotmama.com
Customer Service: 800-217-3750
Clothing, nursing, baby gear.

One Step Ahead 📖
Website: http://www.onestepahead.com
Customer Service: 800-274-8440
Clothing, baby care, gear, safety, pregnancy, and more.

Parent to be Calendar
Website: http://www.2bparent.com/calendar
Customer Service: 954-782-8668 Fax: 954-782-9656
Parenting and pregnancy videos.

Pregnant Inc.
Website: http://www.pregnantinc.com
Customer Service: 626-288-6220
Bedding, furniture, and baby gear.

Pregnancy
Website: http://www.women.com/pregnancy
Customer Service: online form
Parenting, pregnancy, babycare, and safety.

Pregnancy
Website: http://www.pregnancy.about.com/americanbaby
Customer Service: 212-204-4000
Pregnancy.

Pregnancy Weekly
Website: http://www.pregnancyweekly.com
Customer Service: online form
Pregnancy and baby names.

Pump In Style
Website: http://www.pumpinstyle.com
Customer Service: 877-9-DIAPER Fax: 250-336-8848
Nursing, maternity, baby care, toys, clothing, etc.

Red Calliope
Website: http://www.redcalliope.com
Customer Service: 800-421-0526
Safety, bedding, maternity, and baby care.

Royal Baby
Website: http://www.royalbaby.com
Customer Service: 866-855-1945 Fax: 309-416-4472
Parenting, pregnancy, clothing, toys, gifts, etc.

Sesame Street
Website: http://www.sesamestreet.com
Customer Service: online form
Stories, games, parenting, music, pregnancy, etc.

Sesame Street Workshop
Website: http://www.sesameworkshop.org
Customer Service: online form
Stories, games, parenting, music, pregnancy, etc

Stork Helper Birth Kits
Website: http://www.storkhelper.com
Customer Service: 877-605-4253
Pregnancy kits in case of early delivery.

Sure Baby
Website: http://www.suurebaby.com
Customer Service: customercare@surebaby.com
Pregnancy, gifts, and baby care.

Target Lullaby Club
Website: http://www.target.com
Customer Service: 800-888-9333
Everything baby.

TL Care
Website: http://www.tlcare.com
Customer Service: online form
Baby care, parenting, and nursing products.

Toys R Us
Website: http://www.toysrus.com
Customer Service: 800-TOYS-R-Us
Toys, feeding, baby care, gear,bedding/furniture, books/music.

Twins Magazine
Website: http://www.twinsmagazine.com
Customer Service: 888-558-9467
Twin and pregnancy information.

UK Mother
Website: http://www.ukmother.com
Customer Service: UK
Pregnancy, health, baby gear.

You and Your Child
Website: http://www.tesco.com/youandyourchild
Customer Service: UK
Pregnancy, parenting, feeding, and baby care.

Your Baby Today
Website: http://www.yourbabytoday.com
Customer Service: online form
Pregnancy and parenting.

Zenoff Productions
Website: http://www.zenoffprod.com
Customer Service: pmacomber@zenoffprod.com
Nursing pillows.

Toys, Activities, and Playsets

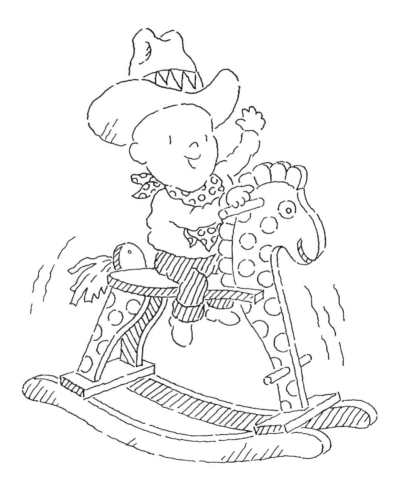

A&A Plush
Website: http://www.aaplush.com
Customer Service: 800-227-5874
Plush toys.

ABC Development Inc.
Website: http://www.abc-development.com
Customer Service: 888-222-3053
Baby care, feeding, and toys.

Able Baby
Website: http://www.ablebaby.com
Customer Service: ablebabyco@aol.com
Safety, baby care, bedding, books/music/videos, toys.

ADZ Baby Gifts
Website: http://www.adz-baby-gifts.com
Customer Service: 800-464-0042
Clothing, toys, and gift baskets.

Alley Opp Sports.com
Website: http://www.alleyoppsports.com
Customer Service: 877-ALLEY-OOP
Outdoor playsets.

Alternative Baby
Website: http://www.alternativebaby.com
Customer Service: 800-469-1126
Baby care, gear, clothing, pregnancy, toys, and gifts baskets.

American Baby Company
Website: http://www.americanbaby.com
Customer Service: 909-597-9070
Clothing, toys, pregnancy, parenting, and gifts.

American Creative Team, Inc.
Website: http://www.us-act.com
Customer Service: 800-747-5689
Toys and baby room décor.

American Girl 📖
Website: http://www.americangirl.com
Customer Service: 800-845-0005
Toys for girls.

Anatex
Website: http://www.anatex.com
Customer Service: 800-999-9599
Rollercoaster mini mazes.

Arrivals Baby Gifts
Website: http://www.arrivalsbabygifts.com
Customer Service: 800-741-0254
Toys, gifts, and bedding.

A Smart Baby
Website: http://www.asmartbaby.com
Customer Service: 877-310-6647
Toys, gifts, books/videos, and announcements.

Attachments
Website: http://www.attachmentscatalog.com
Customer Service: 800-873-5023
Toys, breastfeeding, gifts, books, and baby gear.

Babies-R-Us
Website: http://www.babiesrus.com
Customer Service: 800-BABYRUS
Everything baby.

Baby Ant
Website: http://www.babyant.com
Customer Service: online form
Toys, clothing, health, bedding, and gifts.

Baby Bargains
Website: http://www.babybargains.com
Customer Service: 540-899-6090
Toys, pregnancy, and clothing.

Baby Bazaar
Website: http://www.babybazaar.com
Customer Service: 877-543-7186
Clothing, baby gear, toys, bedding, and gifts.

Baby Bjorn
Website: http://www.babybjorn.com
Customer Service: 800-593-5522
Baby gear, toys, feeding, and baby care.

Baby Boom
Website: http://www.babyboom1.com
Customer Service: 800-929-4666
Gifts, pregnancy, clothing and toys.

Baby Box
Website: http://babybox.com
Customer Service: 800-373-8216
Boutique baby gifts, books/music, clothing, bedding, and toys.

Baby Bundles
Website: http://www.babybundle.com
Customer Service: 877-620-BABY
Toys and games.

Baby Bunz
Website: http://www.babybunz.com
Customer Service: 800-676-4559 Fax: 360-354-1203
Baby care, clothing, bedding, toys, books, feeding.

Baby Care
Website: http://babycare-sa.com
Customer Service: 866-343-2836
Baby gear, bedding, gifts, nursing, toys, and more.

Baby Catalog of America
Website: http://www.babycatalog.com
Customer Service: 800-PLAYPEN
Baby gear, furniture, baby care, toys, and feeding.

Baby Catalogue, The 📖
Website: http://www.thebabycatalogue.com
Customer Service: London
Clothing, feeding, baby care, gear, bedding, safety, and toys.

Baby Corner, The
Website: http://www.thebabycorner.com
Customer Service: 812-867-3759
Baby care, gear, pregnancy, parenting, clothing, toys, bedding.

Baby Cyberstore
Website: http://www.babycyberstore.com
Customer Service: 757-369-0254 Fax: 757-369-0256
Bedding, toys, baby gear, and feeding.

Baby Emporio
Website: http://www.babyemporio.com
Customer Service: 800-965-9909
Ookie and Kammi dolls, blankets and soothys.

Baby Gift Place
Website: http://www.babygiftplace.com
Customer Service: 800-333-5690
Toys and gifts.

Baby Heirlooms
Website: http://www.babyheirlooms.com
Customer Service: 800-340-8838
Toys, clothing, and gifts.

Baby Lane
Website: http://www.thebabylane.com
Customer Service: 888-387-0019
Toys, baby care, and baby gear.

Baby Mountain
Website: http://www.babymountain.com
Customer Service: mail@babymountain.com
Announcements, clothing, feeding, names, toys, safety, bedding.

Baby Navigator
Website: http://www.babynavigator.com
Customer Service: online form
Safety, bedding, feeding, toys, baby care, gear, clothing, books.

Baby Online
Website: http://www.babyonline.com
Customer Service: London
Parenting, baby care, toys, and feeding.

Baby Place
Website: http://www.baby-place.com
Customer Service: online form
Health/safety, parenting, pregnancy, and toys.

Baby Products Online
Website: http://www.babyproductsonline.com
Customer Service: 626-914-9905
Gifts, toys, bedding, and baby gear.

Baby Resource
Website: http://www.babyresource.com
Customer Service: online form
Toys, health/safety, and books/music.

Baby Smart Start
Website: http://www.babysmartstart.com
Customer Service: 919-767-2100 Fax: 919-767-2700
Toys.

Baby Style
Website: http://www.babystyle.com
Customer Service: 877-ESTYLES
Bedding, toys, clothing, baby gear, baby care and gifts.

Baby Supermall
Website: http://www.babysupermall.com
Customer Service: online form
Baby care, feeding, toys, bedding, clothing,safety, and gifts.

Baby Toy Town
Website: http://www.babytoytown.com
Customer Service: 626-288-6220
Toys, bedding, baby gear, and gifts.

Baby Ultimate
Website: http://www.babyultimate.com
Customer Service: 877-724-4537
Clothing and toys.

Baby Universe
Website: http://www.babyuniverse.com
Customer Service: 877-615-BABY Fax: 954-523-9881
Safety, feeding, books/music, baby care, gear, toys, bedding.

Baby's Abode
Website: http://www.babysabode.com
Customer Service: 866-4BBABODE
Toys, baby care, and bedding.

Baby's Heaven
Website: http://www.babysheaven.com
Customer Service: 866-343-2836
Toys, bedding, health/safety, baby care, gear, gifts.

Babyking 📖
Website: http://babyking.com
Customer Service: 800-424-BABY
Toys, feeding, clothing, baby care, and gifts.

Babynet Center
Website: http://www.babynetcenter.com
Customer Service: online form
Books/music, clothing, feeding, bedding, toys, baby gear.

Babyworks
Website: http://www.babyworks.com
Customer Service: 800-422-2910
Feeding, toys, babycare, bedding, clothing.

Backyard Adventures
Website: http://www.backyardadventures.com
Customer Service: 859-296-1361
Outdoor playsets.

Backyard Enterprises, Inc.
Website: http://www.backyardenterprises.com
Customer Service: 800-345-1491
Outdoor playsets.

Barbie
Website: http://www.barbie.com
Customer Service: 800-432-KIDS
Barbie dolls.

Barclay Woods
Website: http://www.barclaywoods.com
Customer Service: 877-385-6760
Toys.

Barney for Baby
Website: http://www.barneyforbaby.com
Customer Service: 800-418-2371
Barney clothing, books, music, toys, gifts, etc.

Bareware
Website: http://bareware.net
Customer Service: 877-9 DIAPER
Clothing, toys, baby care, gear, and pregnancy.

Battat
Website: http://www.battat-toys.com
Customer Service: 800-247-6144 / 800-822-8828
Toys.

Bob the Builder
Website: http://www.bobthebuilder.com
Customer Service: 888-427-0720
Bob the Builder everything - clothing, bedding, toys, books, etc.

Brio Toys
Website: http://www.briotoys.com
Customer Service: 888-274-6869
Toys.

Canada Baby Works
Website: http://www.canadababyworks.com
Customer Service: 877-531-BABY
Clothing, baby care, gear, toys, and pregnancy.

Cedar Works
Website: http://www.cedarworks.com
Customer Service: 800-GO-CEDAR
Outdoor playsets.

Cherished Moments
Website: http://www.cherishedmoments.com
Customer Service: 713-957-2764 Fax: 713-957-2764
Toys, bedding, parenting, names, and baby gear.

Chicco USA
Website: http://www.chiccousa.com
Customer Service: 877-424-4226
Baby gear and toys.

Child Life
Website: http://www.childlife.com
Customer Service: 800-GO-SWING
Outdoor playsets.

Childcraft Education
Website: http://www.childcraft.com
Customer Service: 800-631-5652
Toys.

Children's Orchard
Website: http://www.childorch.com
Customer Service: 800-999-KIDS
Baby gear, toys, and clothing.

Comfort Living
Website: http://www.baby-store.net
Customer Service: 877-378-4411
Feeding, health/safety, baby gear, bedding, toys, pregnancy.

Company Store, The
Website: http://www.thecompanystore.com
Customer Service: 800-323-8000
Toys, bedding, clothing, and baby care.

Cookie Baby Inc.
Website: http://www.cookiebabyinc.com
Customer Service: 877-787-0088
Personalized baby products. Toys, bedding and gifts.

Cosco Inc.
Website: http://www.coscoinc.com
Customer Service: 800-544-1108
Toys and baby gear.

Crayola
Website: http://www.crayola.com
Customer Service: online form
Crayola crayons, pens, and more.

Creative Play Things
Website: http://www.creativeplaythings.com
Customer Service:800-24-SWING
Outdoor playsets

Creativity for Kids
Website: http://www.creativityforkids.com
Customer Service:800-311-8684 ext. 3037
Activities.

Detailed Play
Website: http://www.detailedplay.com
Customer Service: 800-398-7565
Outdoor playsets.

Discovery Toys Inc.
Website: http://www.discoverytoysinc.com
Customer Service: 800-426-4777
Discovery toys.

Disney Interactive
Website: http://www.disneyinteractive.com
Customer Service: 800-688-1520
Games/activites via the website.

Disney Learning
Website: http://www.disneylearning.org
Customer Service: 800-688-1520
Educational play.

Disney Playhouse
Website: http://www.playhousedisney.com
Customer Service: 800-688-1520
Games/activites via the website.

Dragon Fly Toys
Website: http://www.dragonflytoys.com
Customer Service: 800-308-2208 Fax: 204-453-2320
Toys and books.

E Baby Station
Website: http://ebabystation.com
Customer Service: 706-863-4452 Fax: 706-863-4452
Bedding, gifts, pregnancy, baby care, gear, clothing, and toys.

E Baby Superstore
Website: http://www.ebabysuperstore.com
Customer Service: 877-253-7717 Fax: 425-357-1856
Toys, safety, baby care, baby gear, books/music..

EStyle
Website: http://www.estyle.com
Customer Service: 877-ESTYLES
Bedding, toys, clothing, pregnancy, gifts, and baby gear.

E Toys
Website: http://www.etoys.com
Customer Service: 888-753-5568
Toys.

Educo
Website: http://www.educo.com
Customer Service: 800-661-4142
Bead and wire mazes (educational toys).

First Toys
Website: http://www.firsttoys.com
Customer Service: 800-210-7318
Toys, books, and music.

First Years, The
Website: http://www.thefirstyears.com
Customer Service: 800-325-5088
Toys

Fisher Price
Website: http://www.fisher-price.com
Customer Service: 800-432-5437
Toys.

Folk Manis 📖
Website: http://www.folkmanis.com
Customer Service: 800-654-8922
Outdoor playsets.

Funny Friends
Website: http://www.funnyfriends.com
Customer Service: 877-45FUNNY
Plush toys.

Genius Baby
Website: http://www.geniusbaby.com
Customer Service: 704-573-4500 Fax: 704-545-5716
Baby gifts, books and toys.

Gifts for Baby
Website: http://www.giftsforbaby.com
Customer Service: 201-493-8722
Clothing, toys, and gifts.

Great Beginnings
Website: http://www.childrensfurniture.com
Customer Service: 800-886-7099
Bedding/furniture, baby gear, toys, safety, books/music, and gifts.

Gund
Website: http://www.gund.com
Customer Service: 800-448-4863
Toys.

Hart Toys
Website: http://www.harttoys.com
Customer Service: 800-859-HART Fax: 360-693-7811
Toys.

Hasbro
Website: http://www.hasbro.com
Customer Service: 888-836-7025
Toys.

Haystack Toys
Website: http://www.haystacktoys.com
Customer Service: 877-I-INVENT
Toys.

Hedscape
Website: http://www.hedscape.com
Customer Service: 800-323-5999
Toys, gymsets, and trampolines.

Imaginarium
Website: http://www.imaginarium.com
Customer Service: 88-TOYOLOGY
Toys, books, and music.

Imagiix
Website: http://www.imagiix.com
Customer Service: 800-IMAGIIX
Toys.

Infantino
Website: http://www.infantino.com
Customer Service: 800-365-8182 Fax: 858-457-0181
Toys, bedding, and baby gear.

International Playthings
Website: http://www.intplay.com
Customer Service: 800-631-1272
Toys.

KB Kids
Website: http://www.kbkids.com
Customer Service: 877-5KBTOYS
Toys.

KB Toys
Website: http://www.kbtoys.com
Customer Service: 877-5KBTOYS
Toys.

Kid Toy Shop
Website: http://www.kidtoyshop.com
Customer Service: 888-545-9393 Fax: 888-447-9088
Toys.

Kidology Toys
Website: http://www.kidologytoys.com
Customer Service: 800-995-4436 Fax: 800-995-0506
Educational site.

Kids II
Website: http://www.kidsii.com
Customer Service: 770-751-0442
Toys, bedding, baby care, and baby gear.

Klutz
Website: http://www.klutz.com
Customer Service: 800-737-4123
Books and toys

Lamaze Learning Curve
Website: http://www.lamaze.com
Customer Service: online form
Toys.

Lamaze Toys
Website: http://www.lamazetoys.com
Customer Service: 800-704-8697 Fax: 312-981-7500
Educational/manipulative toys.

Lawn Toys
Website: http://www.lawntoys.com
Customer Service: 800-827-7858
Toys.

Leap Frog
Website: http://www.leapfrog.com
Customer Service: 800-701-LEAP
Books and educational toys.

Learning Curve
Website: http://www.learningcurve.com
Customer Service: 800-704-8697
Educational toys.

Lego
Website: http://www.lego.com
Customer Service: 800-453-4652 Fax: 888-FAX-LEGO
Toys.

Lillian Vernon Kids
Website: http://www.lillianvernon.com
Customer Service: 800-285-555
Toys and gifts - personalization available.

Little Tikes
Website: http://www.littletikes.com
Customer Service: 800-321-0183
Toys.

Lizzie's Looking Glass
Website: http://www.lizzieslookingglass.com
Customer Service: 888-545-9393
Educational toys.

Luv n' Care
Website: http://www.luvncare.com
Customer Service: 888-LUVNCARE
Baby care, toys, and bedding.

Main Street Toys
Website: http://www.manhattantoys.com
Customer Service: 800-410-2822 Fax: 785-227-4744
Toys.

Manhattan Baby Toys
Website: http://www.manhattanbaby.com
Customer Service: 800-541-1345
Toys.

Mattel
Website: http://www.mattel.com
Customer Service: 800-524-TOYS
Toys.

Meijer Baby Club
Website: http://www.meijer.com/babyclub
Customer Service: 800-543-3704
Feeding, baby gear, bedding, baby care, pregnancy, and toys.

Mr. Potato Head
Website: http://www.mrpotatohead.com
Customer Service: 800-255-5516
Toys

Museum Tour
Website: http://www.museumtour.com
Customer Service: 800-360-9116
Books, music, games, puzzles and creative play.

My First Games
Website: http://www.myfirstgames.com
Customer Service: 800-255-5516
Games

Neat Stuff Gifts
Website: http://www.neatstuffgifts.com
Customer Service: 800-586-9278 Fax: 732-846-9796
Gifts, toys, and bedding.

Nick Jr.
Website: http://www.nickjr.com
Customer Service: Online form
Games, toys, books, videos, etc.

Nickelodeon
Website: http://www.nick.com
Customer Service: Online form
Games, toys, books, videos, etc.

Nickelodeon
Website: http://www.nickelodeon.com
Customer Service: Online form
Games, toys, books, videos, etc.

Nursery Rhymes
Website: http://www.nurseryrhymes.com
Customer Service: 519-743-1321 Fax: 519-743-1681
Baby gear, furniture/bedding, toys, and safety.

Pamela Drake
Website: http://www.woodkins.com
Customer Service: 800-966-3762
Toys and puzzles.

Parent Hub
Website: http://www.parenthub.com
Customer Service: info@parenthub.com
Parenting, clothing, furniture, toys, and books.

Parenting Concepts
Website: http://www.parentingconcepts.com
Customer Service: 800-727-3683
Baby gear, books/music, parenting, toys, and gifts.

PBS Kids
Website: http://www.pbskids.org
Customer Service: 703-739-5000
Parenting and games.

Pecoware
Website: http://www.pecoware.com
Customer Service: 800-456-7326
Toys.

Peg Perego
Website: http://www.perego.com
Customer Service: 800-728-2108
Baby gear and toys.

Playdoh
Website: http://www.playdoh.com
Customer Service: 800-255-5516
Toys.

Playmobil
Website: http://www.playmobil.com
Customer Service: 800-752-9662
Toys.

Playnation 📖
Website: http://www.playset.com
Customer Service: 800-445-PLAY Fax: 770-424-3335
Outdoor playsets.

Playskool
Website: http://www.playskool.com
Customer Service: online form
Toys.

Preemie Store and More, The 📖
Website: http://www.preemie.com
Customer Service: 800-755-4852
Preemie clothing.

Puffer Belly Toys
Website: http://www.pufferbellytoys.com
Customer Service: 877-302-5706
Toys.

Pump In Style
Website: http://www.pumpinstyle.com
Customer Service: 877-9-DIAPER Fax: 250-336-8848
Nursing, maternity, baby care, toys, clothing, etc.

R R Gifts 📖
Website: http://www.rrgifts.com/thomas.html
Customer Service: 888-RRGIFTS
Toys, books, videos, bedding, clothing, and more.

Radio Flyer
Website: http://www.radioflyer.com
Customer Service: 800-621-7613
Wagons and accessories.

Rainbow Play Systems, Inc.
Website: http://www.rainbowplay.com
Customer Service: 800-RAINBOW
Outdoor playsets.

Rich Frog 📖
Website: http://www.richfrog.com
Customer Service: webinfo@richfrog.com
Toys, gifts, and baby care.

Rocking Horse Dreams
Website: http://www.rocking-horse-dreams.com
Customer Service: 877-72-HORSE
Toys.

Royal Baby
Website: http://www.royalbaby.com
Customer Service: 866-855-1945 Fax: 309-416-4472
Parenting, pregnancy, clothing, toys, gifts, etc.

Roylco 📖
Website: http://www.roylco.com
Customer Service: 800-362-8656
Art materials.

Rumpus
Website: http://www.rumpus.com
Customer Service: 212-463-9869 Fax: 212-463-8267
Toys and games.

Russ Berrie & Company
Website: http://www.russberrie.com
Customer Service: 800-358-8278
Plush toys, gifts and bedding accessories.

Sammy's Street Strollers
Website: http://www.streetstrollers.com
Customer Service: 209-274-6110 Fax: 209-274-0862
Pedal car toys.

Sassy
Website: http://www.sassybaby.com
Customer Service: 800-323-6336
Toys, baby care, feeding, and baby gear.

Sesame Street
Website: http://www.sesamestreet.com
Customer Service: online form
Stories, games, parenting, music, pregnancy, etc.

Sesame Street Workshop
Website: http://www.sesameworkshop.org
Customer Service: online form
Stories, games, parenting, music, pregnancy, etc.

Shopping Galore
Website: http://www.shopinggalore.com/Babiesgalore.html
Customer Service: 866-517-9608 Fax: 662-513-6667
Toys, gifts, and much more.

Small World Toys
Website: http://www.smallworldtoys.com
Customer Service: 800-421-4153
Toys.

Sno-Toys
Website: http://www.sno-toys.com
Customer Service: 800-827-7858
Snow toys.

Step 2
Website: http://www.step2company.com
Customer Service: 800-347-8372 Fax: 330-655-9685
Toys.

Sunsational Kids
Website: http://www.sunsationalkids.com
Customer Service: 910-353-6561 Fax: 910-353-5153
Toys, books, music, furniture, and clothing.

Survive The Drive
Website: http://www.survive-the-drive.com
Customer Service: 800-573-6018
Entertainment and travel activities.

TC Timber
Website: http://www.tctimber.com
Customer Service: 800-468-6873
Wooden block toys.

Target Lullaby Club
Website: http://www.target.com
Customer Service: 800-888-9333
Everything baby.

Tangerine Bear
Website: http://www.tangerinebear.com
Customer Service: online form
Videos and toys.

Teddy Luv
Website: http://www.teddyluv.com
Customer Service: 877-HUG-7577
Personalized teddy bear gifts.

Tiny Love
Website: http://www.tinylove.com
Customer Service: 888-TINY-LOVE
Soft developmental toys and magazine.

Tiny Love Store
Website: http://www.tinylovestore.com
Customer Service: 800-843-6292
Soft developmental toys.

Toddler Toys
Website: http://www.toddlertoys.com
Customer Service: online form
Toys.

Tomy
Website: http://www.tomy.co.uk
Customer Service: UK
Educational/manipulative toys.

Tonka Toys
Website: http://www.tonka.com
Customer Service: online form
Toys.

Toon Disney
Website: http://www.disney.com/toon
Customer Service: online form
Games and activities. Everything Disney.

Toy Mobile
Website: http://www.toymobile.com
Customer Service: 888-456-TOYS
Toys

Toynado
Website: http://www.toynado.com
Customer Service: 877-531-2229
Toys.

Toys
Website: http://www.toys.com
Customer Service: 877-452-5437
Toys.

Toys R Us
Website: http://www.toysrus.com
Customer Service: 800-TOYS-R-Us
Toys, feeding, baby care, gear,bedding/furniture, books/music.

Travel Tots
Website: http://www.traveltots.com
Customer Service: 800-205-4144
Travel kits for tots.

Tuttibella
Website: http://www.tuttibella.com
Customer Service: 877-279-9391
Bedding, furniture, clothes, toys, baby gear, and more.

Urban Baby
Website: http://www.urbanbaby.com
Customer Service: online form
Clothing and toys.

W J Fantasy Publishing
Website: http://www.wjfantasy
Customer Service: 800-222-7529
Books and toys.

Waldorf Toys
Website: http://www.waldorf-toys.com
Customer Service: info@waldorf-toys.com
Toys.

Walt Disney
Website: http://www.waltdisney.com
Customer Service: 800-217-7738 ext. 1
Disney items.

Yahoo
Website: http://shoppingyahoo.com
Customer Service: online form
Furniture, clothing, bedding, baby gear, and more.

Zany Brainy
Website: http://www.zanybrainy.com
Customer Service: 877-WOW-KIDS
Toys and books.

Index

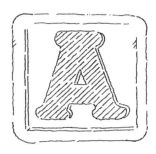

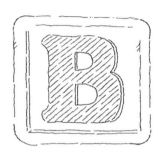

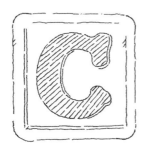

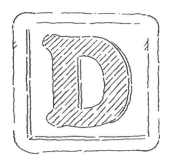

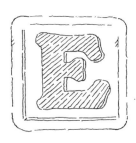

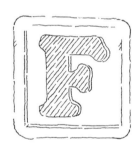

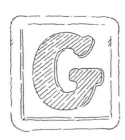

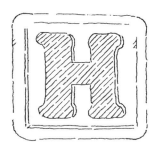

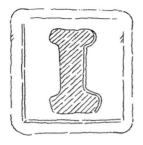

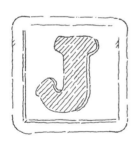

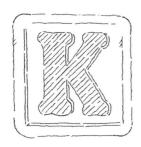

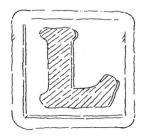

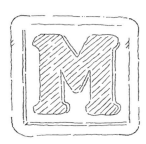

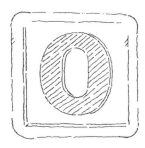

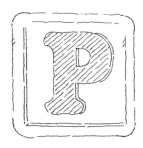

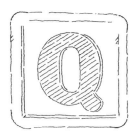

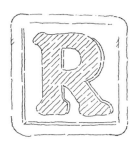

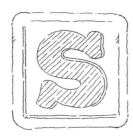

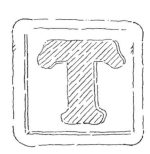

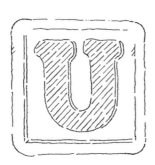

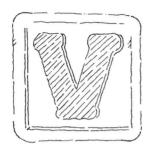

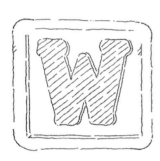

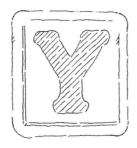

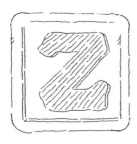

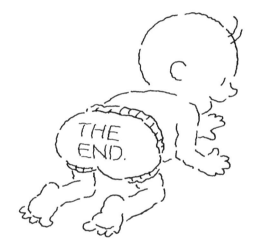

Order Form for The Baby Web book

Would you like more copies of The Baby Web for a friend with a new baby or for a baby shower gift?

Shipping is $3.95 for each book. FREE shipping on orders of two or more books to the same address within the United States.

Order by phone. Have your credit card information ready. 859-879-1892
Order on the Web. http://www.thebabywebbook.com
Order by email. books@chestnutlanedesign.com
Order by mail. Use the order form below, a copy of it, or just simply write your information on a plain piece of paper and mail to:
Chestnut Lane Design, LLC, The Baby Web,
P.O. Box 1039, Versailles, KY 40383.

Send me ____ copies @ $18.95 each = _____
KY residents add 6% sales tax ($1.14 per book) + _____
Subtotal = _____
For 1 book, add $3.95 shipping. For 2 or more books
  to the same address, add $0, shipping is free. + _____
Outside of the Unites States, call for shipping costs.
Total = _____

Make check or money order payable to "Chestnut Lane Design." Or use credit card:
  ☐ Visa   ☐ Mastercard ☐ Discover ☐American Express
Card Number: _____

Epiration date:___/___ Name on card: _____
Authorized Signature: _____

Name:_____
Address: _____
City: _____ State: _____ Zip: _____
Email: _____
Phone Number: (_____)_____
Thank you for your order.